OUT IN THE RURAL

Out in the Rural

A MISSISSIPPI HEALTH CENTER

AND ITS WAR ON POVERTY

Thomas J. Ward Jr.
with a foreword by H. Jack Geiger

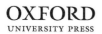

OXFORD
UNIVERSITY PRESS

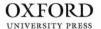

OXFORD
UNIVERSITY PRESS

Oxford University Press is a department of the University of Oxford. It furthers
the University's objective of excellence in research, scholarship, and education
by publishing worldwide. Oxford is a registered trade mark of Oxford University
Press in the UK and certain other countries.

Published in the United States of America by Oxford University Press
198 Madison Avenue, New York, NY 10016, United States of America.

Library of Congress Cataloging-in-Publication Data
Names: Ward, Thomas J., Jr., 1969- author.
Title: Out in the rural : a Mississippi health center and
its war on poverty / Thomas J. Ward Jr.
Description: Oxford ; New York : Oxford University Press, [2016] |
Includes bibliographical references and index.
Identifiers: LCCN 2016021267 (print) | LCCN 2016021721 (ebook) |
ISBN 9780190624620 (hardback : alk. paper) | ISBN 9780190624637 (ebook) |
ISBN 9780190624644 (ebook)
Subjects: | MESH: Geiger, Jack, 1925- | Tufts-Delta Health Center (Mound
Bayou, Miss.) | Community Health Centers—history | Community Health
Services—history | Rural Health Services—history | Social Determinants
of Health—history | Socioeconomic Factors—history | History,
20th Century | Mississippi
Classification: LCC RA395.M627 (print) | LCC RA395.M627 (ebook) |
NLM WA 11 AM7 | DDC 362.1209762—dc23
LC record available at https://lccn.loc.gov/2016021267

9 8 7 6 5 4 3 2

Printed by Sheridan Books, Inc., United States of America

For those whose road led them to Mound Bayou:
Dr. H. Jack Geiger
Dr. John Hatch
Dr. L.C. Dorsey
Dr. Andrew James

Contents

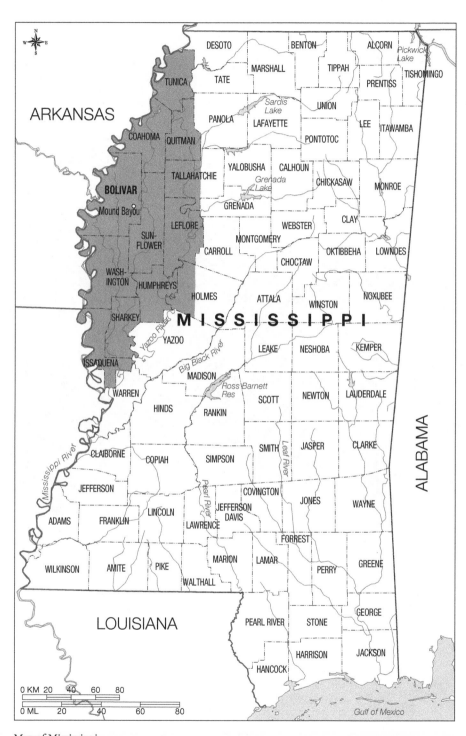

Map of Mississippi

Shaded area indicates Mississippi's Delta Region.

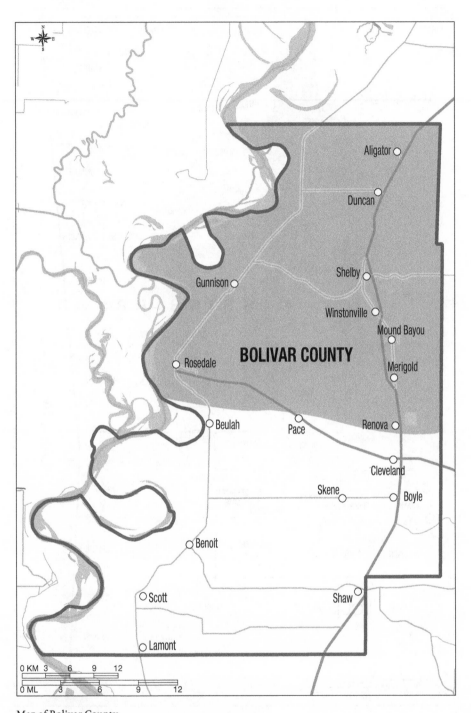

Map of Bolivar County

Shaded area indicates region served by the Tufts–Delta Health Center.

Foreword

THE ANTHROPOLOGIST MARGARET Mead once warned that no one should ever underestimate the ability of a small and determined group of people to change the world. That description surely matches the architects of the contemporary community health center model and its core discipline: community-oriented primary care. Drs. Sidney and Emily Kark, Guy Steuart, John Cassel, and others responded to a small window of opportunity in the early 1940s in—of all places—apartheid South Africa. They launched that first great experiment in a profoundly impoverished and disease-burdened rural "Zulu tribal reserve" named Pholela in South Africa's Natal province. This would be one of the grandfathers of the experiment launched decades later and half a world away in Mississippi and described so dramatically by historian Thomas J. Ward in this book. Today, there are community health centers in forty-two nations across the globe, linked in a recently created International Federation. They vary widely, depending on the political economies and national healthcare systems of their various nations: some with national health services and universal coverage, others with mixed public–private healthcare systems, and some with no coherent healthcare system at all. All of them, however, are committed to a core principle: that community health centers have a dual responsibility, to care not only for the diagnosis and treatment of the individual patients who enter their doors, but also to address the health status of the populations and communities they serve and out of which those patients come. It is fair to say that the Karks and their successors have changed the world of healthcare on a global scale.

The American experiment has, similarly, undergone explosive growth over the half century since its initiation in Mississippi and Boston in 1965. In the United States, there are now more than 1,300 community health centers, delivering primary care at more than 9,000 sites of clinical service and providing care to an estimated 28 million low-income and minority patients. These centers are both urban and rural; some are located in the three great streams of migrant farm workers in the United States, while others serve students in public high schools, residents of public housing projects, or more than one million homeless men, women, and children—families in desperate need of care. (Today, twenty-one such health centers are in Mississippi.) These new models of care also have varied widely from one another, and over time, in the degree to which they have successfully intervened in population health status.

The Mississippi experiment described in these pages tested a bold hypothesis—that a community health center can serve as an instrument of social change, intervening not only in the social determinants of its population's health but also launching a process of structural change that starts to liberate that population, through community empowerment, from repetitive cycles of poverty and political exclusion. The Tufts–Delta Health Center fused the two long-separated disciplines of clinical care and public health. It directly addressed problems of hunger and malnutrition, deteriorating housing, unsafe water, primitive sanitation, inferior education, and political isolation and powerlessness. To do so the health center assembled a staff extending well beyond the usual array of essentially clinical personnel—physicians, dentists, nurses, nurse midwives, pharmacists, psychologists, and technicians. To these it added community organizers, environmental engineers, social workers, sanitarians, health educators, agricultural experts, and lawyers. Its most important tool in these efforts was slow, patient, community organization, rooted in the belief that even poor, largely unemployed, often poorly educated, politically oppressed and socially isolated people and communities had within themselves the intelligence, resilience, and determination to confront those problems and create significant change. The ultimate goal was to establish pathways out of poverty and into a better life.

And so, as this book describes, in addition to all the conventional elements of primary clinical care the Tufts–Delta Health Center dug safe wells, built sanitary privies, repaired housing unfit for human habitation, wrote and filled prescriptions for food in crisis situations, and organized a 500-acre cooperative farm, which drew on the agricultural knowledge and skills of its target population, producing thousands of tons of vegetables and helping to reduce local malnutrition. It also undertook extensive educational and training programs of its own. In all of these efforts, the target population remained fully engaged, and each community set its own priorities.

As Thomas Ward's vivid and meticulously researched account makes clear, the health center's efforts rested on three pillars of strength. The first was the civil rights movement itself—the years of brave, nonviolent, and determined efforts by the Student Nonviolent Coordinating Committee (SNCC), the Congress of Racial Equality (CORE), and the Southern Christian Leadership Conference (SCLC) to accomplish voter registration and directly confront Mississippi's racial caste system. Their work was ultimately embodied in the passage of the Civil Rights Act and Voting Rights Act of the mid-1960s. A second pillar was the creation of a new federal agency, the Office of Economic Opportunity (OEO), or "War on Poverty," committed to a bottom-up philosophy of working with the poor rather than a top-down method of informing the poor what was good for them and then funding it. And finally, the health center drew on the strength of a remarkably committed medical school and university, fully supportive of its efforts, which made possible effective recruitment of staff and a high degree of insulation from local political pressures and opposition.

That is not to say, of course, that all this was accomplished seamlessly and without struggle. The health center and its work were fiercely opposed from the very beginning by all the elements of Mississippi's white power structure: its governor, its legislature, its FBI-like "state sovereignty commission," its two United States Senators, their counterparts on county and municipal levels, and by most of Mississippi's medical, hospital, and public health establishments and agencies. Those struggles are a central and important part of this history, along with the relatively neglected topic of social class and political conflict within minority communities when power, elite status, and control of funding become real issues.

Together with the advent of major new national social programs, such as Medicare, Medicaid, and food stamps, there is no question that the health center's work changed the health status of its target population, the roughly 12,000 African-American residents of North Bolivar County. By such standard metrics as fetal losses, infant mortality rates, the incidence of infectious disease, and the successful management of prevalent chronic illnesses such as heart disease, hypertension, and diabetes. For individual patients, increased knowledge, relief of suffering, and access to quality health care reduced the toll of disease. And over and over again, the health center literally saved the lives of black infants and children. The North Bolivar County Health and Civic Improvement Association, chartered to address issues beyond individual personal medical services, has for decades now owned and operated the nonprofit Delta Health Center as the recipient of its federal grants and other major sources of revenue. It has managed so successfully that the Delta Health Center currently has new state-of-the-art clinical facilities and satellite branches in

four other Delta counties. The health center itself remains a major source of employment and an economic engine for growth in Bolivar County.

There is another dimension to these accomplishments—less tangible but, I believe, as important as any of the others. It is eloquently summarized in a single
phrase by John Hatch, the community organizer described by Tom Ward as "the
soul of the project," to an interviewer from Chronicles, a website that attempts to
tell the histories of all of the community health centers in the United States. "We
changed their dreams," John Hatch said. In what he called "The Prep Academy,"
the health center opened its own Office of Education and launched its own education and training programs, ranging from high school equivalency certifications
(GED) to pre-college and pre-professional courses taught by the center's own professional staff. In addition, local staff recruits were sent off to other OEO training
programs in Arkansas and Tennessee to produce medical record librarians, secretaries, mid-level administrators, and technicians. Finally, as part of the heady national
atmosphere of civil rights expansion, the health center's professional staff—often
imploring their own alma maters—arranged admissions to prep schools, colleges,
and professional schools across the nation, creating pathways to higher education
from which the African-American people of Bolivar County had long been isolated.
They produced black physicians, nurses, dentists, social workers, psychologists, environmental engineers and business managers on a scale not previously imagined.

These were critical pathways out of poverty. They changed the aspirations—the
dreams—of adults and children alike. For a population largely unemployed, displaced by the mechanization of cotton agriculture, but increasingly determined to
find a road out and change the very structure of their society, this was perhaps the
project's most important impact. John Hatch has lost count, but we know that there
are more than a hundred Bolivar County African Americans now employed in the
health sector alone in Mississippi and other Southern states at every level from tech-
nician to physician. (On his last visit back to the health center Dr. Andrew James,
the director of the project's environmental programs, met the young black high
school graduate who had served as his secretary and administrative assistant in the
1960s. She had come to introduce him to her daughter, a pediatrician.) These interventions, I believe, were the greatest levers of change, for they flowed downward over
time into successive generations, dreaming bigger dreams and living better lives.

The Delta Health Center experiment teaches us that structural change is possible, and that community health centers and allied institutions have a role to play
in it. But this glass is only half full. Racism, residential segregation, segregated
and inferior schools, and attempts at voter suppression still exist, as do the great
toxic concentrations of poverty in urban ghettos. Full-scale urban equivalents
of this Mississippi experiment remain to be invented. They will likely take the

form of interprofessional and multiple agency collaboration, and health personnel working in nongovernmental organizations as well as in clinical care. Such efforts stand on strong shoulders of precedent. Pediatricians led the campaign to end child labor in the United States. Physicians helped to draft this nation's first tenement laws, establishing baseline standards of space, air, and density for the housing of the poor.

More than 200 years ago Johann Peter Franck, the Austrian dean of an Italian medical school delivered a scathing commencement address directly linking the cruelty of social and political structures to the brutally stunted lives and early deaths of the poor. He called his talk "The People's Misery: Mother of All Disease." The attempt to meet that challenge, exemplified in this small corner of a rural county in Mississippi, remains to be completed. This book tells us that this is not, after all, an impossible dream.

H. Jack Geiger, MD

Acknowledgments

I WOULD NOT have had the opportunity to be a part of this wonderful story had it not been for Professor John Dittmer, the Bancroft-award winning historian of Mississippi, who contacted me at the end of 2011 to inquire whether I would be interested in collaborating with Dr. H. Jack Geiger on a history of the Tufts–Delta Health Center. At the time I was working on a book on black prisoners of war, just had been named chair of my department, had young children at home, and had absolutely no interest in starting any new project. However, a call from Professor Dittmer, the author of *Local People* and one of the real giants in the field of both Southern history and African-American history, was not something I could ignore.

John told me that he had been helping Jack Geiger, John Hatch, and L.C. Dorsey revise a manuscript that they had been working on for years about their experiences founding and running the Tufts–Delta Health Center. John had met Jack Geiger while working on his book, *The Good Doctors*, and he knew L. C. Dorsey through her work in the civil rights movement in Mississippi. Indeed, Dittmer's interest in this story was much more than just academic; he had known a number of the health center's leading figures for decades, back to his time teaching at Jackson's tiny Tougaloo College, and his own involvement in Mississippi's civil rights struggle. I had met John a couple of times, and he had been an outside reader of my dissertation, but I was incredibly flattered that he would even think of me to work on this project, which held such personal importance to him. When the manuscript was eventually completed, Professor Dittmer read it carefully and provided me with invaluable insights. I am in debt to him for both the opportunity to get involved in this project and the assistance he provided in bringing it to fruition.

Dittmer said that although he had agreed to help Geiger, Hatch, and Dorsey revise their manuscript, titled "Three Roads to Mound Bayou," he (and they) eventually realized that the project needed much more than revision. To do the story of the Tufts–Delta Health Center justice, a more complete treatment from a professional historian was necessary. Dittmer, recently retired from DePauw University, contacted me, because of my background in Mississippi and African-American health-care history, to see if I would be interested in working on the project. Needless to say, he convinced me, and a couple of weeks later Jack Geiger flew to Mobile to talk about the project and how we would proceed.

Jack Geiger, whom John Dittmer described to me as "one of my heroes," is one of the most remarkable human beings I have ever met. When I first met Jack he was well into his eighties, battling a number of health issues, yet still working as a physician in New York, writing articles, and lecturing all over the country. "The Father of Community Health," as he is known, has had a remarkable career as a physician and humanitarian, working for civil rights and health care all over the world. I originally had intended to coauthor this book with Jack, but we soon decided that the best way forward was for me to take over the project, and enlist Jack's input as I progressed. His input, indeed, proved vital to the completion of this book. He sent me boxes of his personal papers (which will eventually be housed in the Southern Historical Collection at the University of North Carolina–Chapel Hill), provided invaluable commentary, and went through each line of the manuscript, editing it for both content and style. Jack even spent a week in the archives with me in North Carolina, meticulously going through documents. The staff at the Wilson Library at UNC were a tremendous help to me during my numerous visits to Chapel Hill. Many of the photos in the book are located in the collection at Chapel Hill, and most were taken by Dan Bernstein, whose family graciously allowed them to be used here. Victor Schoenbach, an old friend of Jack's, helped with some of the photos in the book, lifting them from a film, also titled *Out in the Rural*, made about the health center in 1969.

Jack also introduced me to a number of the people who were central to the establishment of the Tufts–Delta Health Center, especially John Hatch, who provided vital insights to the creation of the health center, especially the farm co-op and the health council, areas with which he was intimately involved. In addition to John Hatch, a host of other figures of the Tufts–Delta Health Center were generous in allowing me to interview them, or in providing me materials on the health center, especially L. C. Dorsey, Aaron Shirley, Robert Smith, Andrew James, Helen Barnes, Anne Haendel, and Sarah Atkinson. John Fairman, the current director of the Delta Health Center, showed me great hospitality in making sure that I was invited to all the special events commemorating the founding of the center.

Before I became involved with this project, Jack Geiger had secured grant funding from the Ford Foundation, the Robert Wood Johnson Foundation, the Ryan Community Health Network (RCHN) Community Health Foundation, and the Geiger-Gibson Program to tell the story of the Tufts–Delta Health Center. I was the beneficiary of these funds in both direct and indirect ways; much of the work done by Geiger and Dittmer before I came on board was funded by these grants, as were my own travels to Mississippi and North Carolina. Professor Sara Rosenbaum of the Milken Institute School of Public Health at George Washington University administered the grants, and I am grateful to her and her staff, Shelia West and Tishra Beeson, for all their assistance in getting me the funding needed to complete this project. Jack also put me in touch with our editor at Oxford University Press, Chad Zimmerman, who has worked tirelessly to move this project from manuscript to book in a very short period of time. I am in his debt for all the work he has done on a tight schedule to make this book a reality.

I could not have taken on this project without my background in Mississippi history, which I learned during my time in graduate school at the University of Southern Mississippi. There I was lucky enough to study under Neil R. McMillen, the author of *Dark Journey*, which won the Bancroft prize in 1990 and remains the best book ever written about the state of Mississippi, as well as Charles Bolton, the godfather of oral history in the state. Neither Neil nor Chuck read this manuscript, but their fingerprints are all over it, as virtually everything I know about the history of Mississippi came from them. My time in Hattiesburg also provided me with a cadre of historians who remain close friends and professional confidants to this day, especially Glenn Robins, Kathy Barbier, Karen Cox, Andrew Wiest, Curtis Austin, and Marjorie Spurill.

Finally, I would like to thank all those who have supported me day-in and day-out over the four years that I worked on this book, my family and my colleagues at Spring Hill College. I am blessed to work with a wonderful group of people every day at Spring Hill, especially those in the History Department: Pat Harrison, Sarah Duncan, David Head, Shane Dillingham, David Borbridge, and Neil Hamilton. I also would like to acknowledge my students, in particular my 2016 Senior Seminar class, who served as an informal focus group for this work, and picked out the cover photo. Most importantly, I want to thank my wife, Margaret, and our three boys, Pat, Jack, and Teague, for all their love and support.

A Note on Sources

WHEN I BECAME involved in the project in 2011, after being contacted by Professor John Dittmer, I received boxes of materials that he and Jack Geiger had been collecting for years. Three of the founding members of the Tufts–Delta Health Center—Jack Geiger, John Hatch, and L. C. Dorsey—had been working for almost twenty years assembling their memoirs of the health center in what they envisioned would be chapters in a book. Although I have not used their narratives as they had originally intended, the basis of much of my research came from their writings. In addition, all three of them had assembled a vast array of materials that were invaluable in writing this book, including letters, clippings, documents, audiotapes, and even their own personal notes. As a historian, not having assembled many of the research materials myself, I was a bit overwhelmed as to what to do with materials that others had collected. Where possible, I have tried to give the reader the clearest explanation of where every piece of material came from and where it can be located. At this time, however, many of the materials used for this book remain in my possession. Along with these private sources, a wealth of materials on the Tufts–Delta Health Center can be found in the Delta Health Center Records (Collection 04613) in the Southern Historical Collection at the Wilson Library at the University of North Carolina at Chapel Hill. The personal papers of John Hatch, who became a professor of public health at Chapel Hill following his time in Mound Bayou, are also located in the Southern Historical Collection. The materials I have in my possession will be donated to the Southern Historical Collection as well, so future researchers will have access to the same materials I did in writing this history.

Abbreviations used in the Notes

DHC   Delta Health Center Records, Southern Historical Collection, UNC-Chapel Hill

DFP   Dorothy Ferebee Papers, Moorland-Spingarn Research Center, Howard University, Washington, DC

JHC   John Hatch Collection (private, in possession of the author)

JHP   John Hatch Papers, Southern Historical Collection, UNC–Chapel Hill

JGC   Jack Geiger Collection (private, in the possession of the author)

LCDP   L. C. Dorsey Papers (private, in possession of the author)

MSC   Mississippi Sovereignty Commission files, Mississippi Department of Archives and History, Sovereignty Commission Online (http://mdah.state.ms.us/arrec/digital_archives/sovcom/).

The title *Out in the Rural* is borrowed from a short film of the same name produced in 1969 by Judy Schader Rogers. This 22-minute film about the Tufts–Delta Health Center can be viewed online:

http://www.socialmedicine.org/2008/06/04/community-health/out-in-the-rural-a-health-center-in-mississippi-with-jack-geiger/

OUT IN THE RURAL

Of all the forms of inequality, injustice in health care is the most shocking and inhumane.
MARTIN LUTHER KING JR., 1966

Introduction

THE CIVIL RIGHTS movement in Mississippi coalesced during the summer of 1964, as activists from all over the United States launched an initiative to increase black voter registration across a state where it historically had been suppressed. This volunteer movement, branded *Freedom Summer*, brought hundreds of activists to Mississippi, including a subset of physicians and medical students who organized at the same time to provide health and medical care to activists. This group, composed of black and white physicians from inside and outside Mississippi, called themselves the Medical Committee for Human Rights, or MCHR.

The Medical Committee for Human Rights' initial goals were not limited to providing triage care for Freedom Summer; it sought also to desegregate Southern hospitals and to protest the American Medical Association's (AMA's) continued allowance of its affiliate organizations in the South to exclude black physicians—thereby denying them both AMA membership and many of the privileges that went along with such membership, including continuing education and hospital access. The MCHR, as one member described it, "really became the medical arm of the civil rights movement."[1]

But as the physicians of the MCHR became immersed in the summer of activism in Mississippi, their goals for the organization began to change. Horrified by the

---

[1] John Dittmer, *The Good Doctors: The Medical Committee for Human Rights and the Struggle for Social Justice in Health Care* (New York: Bloomsbury, 2009), xi. "An interview with Robert Smith, M.D." Interviewed by Harriet Tanzman, Tougaloo College Archives, 2000.

conditions that they saw black Mississippians living under as they tromped through
the state on their civil rights activities, they became convinced of the inability to
truly bring about racial equality without dramatic improvements in the health care
of the state's black population. Dr. Bob Smith, a black physician from Jackson and
head of the southern branch of the MCHR, recalled his experience touring the
most rural parts of his own state during that summer:

> I understood for the first time what it truly meant to be black in Mississippi,
> and underprivileged, and poor and without medical care, and saw people
> by the hundreds, and really by the thousands, go without medical care. . . .
> Saw what I call a Third-World country. . . . People had been denied benefits
> under Social Security. People had been denied benefits for welfare. . . . Thirty
> to 40 percent of children had intestinal parasites. . . . The maternal mortality
> rate was out of this world.[2]

Following their experiences that summer, seventeen MCHR physicians met again
in September 1964 at the New York City home of Dr. Sidney Greenberg to collabo-
rate on establishing medical programs for destitute black Mississippians. In their
notes from the meeting, the group stated, "We are deeply concerned with the health
needs of the socially deprived. It is our purpose to initiate activities to improve their
health status and to provide professional support and assistance to organizations
concerned with human rights." Through exhaustive fundraising and local collaboration with the Delta Ministry of the National Council of Churches—a civil rights
organization that operated programs in citizenship, education, and economic development, and provided welfare and relief services in eight Mississippi counties—the
MCHR opened the Mileston Health Clinic in Holmes County, on the southern
edge of the Mississippi Delta region, in 1965. MCHR physicians volunteered time
at the clinic, and the organization hired two public health nurses to staff it. Dr. Bob
Smith recalled that the Mileston Clinic showed him "that there were so many needs
other than what I was trained to render in medical school—social services, legal
services, clean water, [and] food."[3]

Dr. H. Jack Geiger, a white physician from Boston, had raised $23,000 for the
Mileston project, but he, like many of his colleagues, was disappointed by what
his efforts had yielded. "We had started a small clinic staffed by volunteers and
some other efforts to provide local health services," he remembered. "Nothing

---

[2] Bruce Morgan, "Up from Mississippi," *Tufts Medicine* Vol. 62, No. 2 (Spring 2003): 16–25.
[3] Dittmer, *The Good Doctors*, 61–62; Mark Newman, *Divine Agitators: The Delta Ministry and Civil Rights in Mississippi* (Athens: University of Georgia Press, 2004), 35, 178; "An interview with Robert Smith, M.D."

comprehensive, but the need was staggering." He recalled feeling "let down" after the excitement and promise of the summer, as the civil rights activities in the state waned, and felt frustrated by the clinic's inability to adequately fix the health problems of the poor in Mississippi under the auspices of the Delta Ministry.

As a result of this frustration, on December 11, 1964, MCHR physicians again congregated and met with civil rights leaders in Greenville, Mississippi, this time in the hopes of regaining the momentum of Freedom Summer. Bob Smith told the group that something new was needed—something that would address the health needs of the poor from top to bottom. Geiger, who had spent four months of his final year in medical school in 1957 on a Rockefeller Foundation scholarship working and studying in community health centers in black South African townships, suggested that such a program of community health centers—nonprofit, comprehensive care centers that address needs on a local level—also could be instituted in Mississippi.[4]

The timing was fortuitous: Four months before the meeting in Greenville, Congress had passed the Economic Opportunity Act, which appropriated $974 million for a wide variety of programs to improve the lives of America's poor. The act was part of the "War on Poverty" that President Lyndon Johnson had declared during his first State of the Union address on January 8, 1964. Johnson stated that the cause of poverty often lay "in our failure to give our fellow citizens a fair chance to develop their own capacities, in a lack of education and training, in a lack of medical care and housing, in a lack of descent communities in which to live and bring up their children," and called on the people of the "richest Nation on earth" to join him in his efforts to improve the lives of the more than 20 percent of the nation that was then living in poverty.

The Office of Economic Opportunity (OEO) was the agency created to administer the antipoverty programs of President Johnson's "Great Society." Led by a veteran of John F. Kennedy's presidency, Sargent Shriver, the OEO eliminated a great deal of bureaucratic red tape by reporting directly to the president rather than operating through existing agencies—and by bypassing state and local governments whose previous lack of responsiveness to the poor and underprivileged was seen by many in the Johnson administration as part of the problem. Shriver's OEO encompassed programs such as the Job Corps, Head Start, the Neighborhood Youth

---

[4] H. Jack Geiger, "The First Community Health Centers: A Model of Enduring Value," *Journal of Ambulatory Care Management* Vol. 28, No. 4 (October-December 2005): 313–20; Bonnie Lefkowitz, *Community Health Centers: A Movement and the People Who Made it Happen* (New Brunswick, NJ.: Rutgers University Press, 2007), 7; Morissa G. Sobelson, "Participation, Power, and Place: Roots of the Community Health Center Movement" (Honors thesis: Tufts University, 2009), 41–42; Dittmer, *The Good Doctors, xi*, 65; Morgan, "Up from Mississippi," 22.

Corps, the Adult Basic Education Program, and Volunteers in Service to America (VISTA). The centerpiece of the antipoverty program was the Community Action Program (CAP), a brainchild of Sargent Shriver, which would fund a wide variety of community action agencies. These community action agencies emerged as the most controversial aspects of the War on Poverty, especially in the South and major urban areas. President Johnson was initially opposed to the Community Action Program; Shriver recalls the President telling him, "You can't do it! You can't give federal dollars to private agencies. . . . It won't work. . . . You're going to be in terrible trouble . . . and so will I. It's going to be just awful. The people will steal the money. The governors and mayors will hate it. You're just asking for it, Sarge." As a concession to powerful mayors and governors—especially in the South—who resented such unilateral federal reach, OEO grants for state projects could be vetoed by a governor (although programs administered through institutions of higher education were protected from a state veto, a detail that later would become very significant in the history of the Tufts–Delta Health Center).[5] What ensued as a result of these streamlined procedures, according to historian Bonnie Lefkowitz, "was one of the fastest rollouts of a new federal effort on record. The hard-driving Shriver recruited people like himself, often on loan from their 'day' jobs. . . . They played an active role in developing concepts, finding people to implement them, and nurturing the new projects."

Initially, health programs were not a priority of the OEO's antipoverty agenda, only encompassing about 5 percent of its total budget during its first four years. But officials soon realized the direct relationship between poverty and health as they came into direct contact with the poor through programs such as Head Start and the Job Corps. Much as the physicians of MCHR had come to see the need to combat health problems before they could adequately address civil rights inequities, OEO officials saw that until poor peoples' health was improved, the antipoverty programs would be stuck in the mud. Dr. Robert Kalinowski, who later headed the OEO's health service program, recalled that Job Corps and Head Start programs, "made us painfully aware that there was a lot of health-care deficit in the kids they were seeing." Countless candidates in the Job Corps had never seen a doctor or a dentist, and some children in Head Start programs had not been vaccinated and were too weak to learn because of malnutrition and disease. To deal with these issues, local agencies had come into the practice of applying to OEO to fund purchase of medical services from the private sector. This intervention, however, was both expensive

[5] Michael L. Gilette, *Launching the War on Poverty: An Oral History* (New York: Oxford University Press, 2010), xix; Scott Stossel, *Sarge: The Life and Times of Sargent Shriver* (Washington, DC: Smithsonian Books, 2004), 375–376; Lefkowitz, *Community Health* Centers, 4–5.

and inadequate. As one OEO official recalled, "we very quickly decided that if OEO was going to spend any substantial amount of money on health, it would have to be directed to changing the organizational framework through which health services were being delivered to poor people."[6]

Enter the MCHR with a grant proposal to fund a community health center, just as OEO was beginning to see the need for health programs as part of the War on Poverty. Jack Geiger, then a professor at the Harvard School of Public Health, and Dr. Count Gibson, the Chair of the Department of Preventative Medicine at Tufts University Medical School in Boston, became the faces attached to the grant. A native Southerner, Gibson was among the first white physicians to arrive in Mississippi with the MCHR in 1964. He told Geiger that he would push to have Tufts sponsor the center if federal funding could be secured. Geiger then went to William Kissick in the U.S. Surgeon General's office; after ten minutes of listening to Geiger's plan for community health centers, Kissick picked up his phone, called OEO and said, "There is a crazy man in my office and I am sending him over to you." In March of 1965, Geiger met with Sandy Kravitz, Director of Research and Demonstration Programs at OEO, to pitch him the idea for the community health centers. "I described what a community health center was, what the models had been in [South Africa]," Geiger later recalled, "the concept of community health center as an instrument of social change—of intervention in the social, and biological, and physical environments in a basis of community organization and community empowerment." He then requested $30,000 to conduct a feasibility study to see whether such a health center would work in Mississippi. Kravitz denied the request for a $30,000 feasibility study, and instead awarded Geiger and Gibson a $300,000 grant to start working on the health center right away.[7]

Geiger and Gibson then met with leaders at Tufts to convince them to sponsor the health center. What emerged was a plan for Tufts Medical School to use the OEO funding to sponsor two community health centers to serve the needs of the poor—one in an urban ghetto in the North and the other in the rural South. The urban center was to be established at Columbia Point, a 1,200-unit public housing project in Boston, about four miles from the Tufts campus. Geiger and Gibson were purposely vague, however, about where they planned to establish the Southern center.

---

[6] C. G. McDaniel, "Community health centers more than clinics for the poor" *Arizona Republic* (Sept. 5, 1971); Sar A. Levitan, "Healing the Poor in their Back Yard," in Robert M. Hollister, Bernard M. Kramer, and Seymour S. Bellin, Eds. *Neighborhood Health Centers* (Lexington, Mass.: D. C. Health and Co., 1974), 51; Sobelson, "Participation, Power, and Place," 35–36.

[7] Lefkowitz, *Community Health Centers*, 7–8; Dittmer, *The Good Doctors*, 82; Interview with H. Jack Geiger by Robert Korstad and Neil Boothby, April 22, 1992, Southern Rural Poverty Collection (http://dewitt. sanford.duke.edu/wp-content/uploads/2011/09/GEIGER.pdf).

Their initial proposal to OEO did not even specify in which state they planned to locate the Southern center, because they were aware of the opposition among all Southern Congressional delegations to OEO programs—especially any that intended to aid poor blacks—so they tried to sidestep the issues by not designating a specific area. Mississippi, in particular, had fought the establishment of Head Start in the state, and Shriver wanted to avoid further rancor that he feared could doom other, less-controversial, OEO programs. Geiger recalled that "Shriver was so nervous about getting into health activities and about getting into Mississippi, in particular after the Head Start wars . . . [so] I wrote a proposal for a Columbia Point and a southern rural health center as one proposal. The southern rural site was not specified. That could have been any one of thirteen southern states. What that meant was that Shriver did not have to pass the grant through any congressional delegation except Massachusetts."[8]

The tactic worked, and on June 11, 1965, OEO approved a grant of $1.3 million to fund the two centers. According to Geiger, the fact that Tufts Medical School was involved as the sponsor of the centers was critical. "A key factor in overcoming Shriver's anxiety . . . was that there was a major, quality medical school that they were giving this [grant] to. . . . I don't think that it would have gotten started in any other way," he recalled. Gibson added, "[Tufts] was indispensable. There would've been no way to get started without going through the university."[9] It would be the first time that the federal government teamed with a medical school and local communities to provide health care for low-income residents. Gibson would take the point on the urban project, while Geiger would lead the rural Southern center. On December 11, 1965—exactly a year after the meeting in Greenville, and only six months after the funding was approved by OEO—the Columbia Point Health Center (now the Geiger–Gibson Community Health Center) opened in Boston.

Columbia Point had earned a reputation as the city's least attractive place to live. Separated from the rest of Boston by two highways and a railroad line, the community had no shopping center, grocery stores, or doctors' offices. A large municipal garbage dump nearby attracted rats. It was in this environment that Tufts Medical School began the nation's community health center experiment. To house the center, the Housing Authority donated a dozen apartments, rent-free, to be remodeled for health services, with an emergency room, laboratories, an X-ray unit, examination and waiting rooms, and a pharmacy. Tufts medical students assisted the professional staff of physicians, nurses, and social

---

8 Sobelson, "Participation, Power, and Place," 44–45; Interview with Jack Geiger by Korstad and Boothby.

9 Sobelson, "Participation, Power, and Place," 43–44.

workers, who were available seven days a week, night and day. Geiger and Gibson intended Columbia Point to do more than just deliver health services—they wanted it to be the point of the spear in the War on Poverty, intervening in the cycle of helplessness of those who lived there. To do so, they helped organize the Columbia Point Health Association, an independent entity made up of those who lived in the housing project, to marshal the community's residents to bring about change, as well as to inform and advise the health center of the success of its programs. The health association eventually became involved in helping to design and evaluate the center's programs, construct and review its budget, recruit and train staff, and help resolve conflicts. As Geiger said, "What we have tried to do is bring a social cohesion to the neighborhood, and the new experience of being involved in the type of health care they received."[10]

Within its first few months of operation it became clear that Tufts's health center at Columbia Point was making a significant impact on the health and lives of its residents, the majority of whom were on welfare, with an average weekly family income of just $40. One resident later recalled, "Before the health center, we used to have to call up the police when we had a sick child. It was a blessing when this opened up." A feature of the health care system at Columbia Point became known as "family-centered care," in which each family met with a health care team consisting of an internist, pediatrician, community health nurse, social worker, and family health aide. The team members could pool their information to diagnose family health and social problems, and then implement a unique, comprehensive health plan for each family. This system, according to Geiger, "enables us to look for—and try to deal with—family problems, not just individual problems."[11]

As the Columbia Point Health Center proved to be a successful experiment, OEO director Sargent Shriver authorized the expansion of what would become known as Neighborhood—or Community—Health Centers. In the months following the award of the Tufts grant, OEO funded health centers in Denver, Los Angeles, Chicago, and the South Bronx, all as research and demonstration projects involving university medical schools. These centers, under OEO guidelines, were to provide a full range of ambulatory services; a close liaison with other community services; a working relationship with a local hospital, preferably

---

[10] Ralph McGill, "Health in Action Areas," *The Daily Reporter* (Dover, Ohio), April 26, 1967, p. 4; David Haskell, "Pilot Program: Comprehensive Medical Health Program Proven," *The Daily Herald* (Provo, Utah), April 18, 1968, p. 19; United Press International (UPI), "Comprehensive Health Care for the Needy," *The Bridgeport (Conn.) Post*, April 14, 1968, p.12.

[11] Adam Clymer, *Edward M. Kennedy: A Biography* (New York: Harper Perennial, 2000, rpr., 2009), 83; "Comprehensive Health Care for the Needy," *The Bridgeport (Conn.) Post*, April 14, 1968, p.12.

one with an academic affiliation; and participation of the local population in the center's decision-making.[12]

Money soon became an issue, in part because the OEO's authorizing legislation had not specifically provided any funding for health centers. With the escalation of the war in Vietnam squeezing both the funding and support for the War on Poverty, Shriver decided to call in one of his allies in the Senate to shore up support: his brother-in-law Ted Kennedy. In August 1966 Kennedy toured Columbia Point, observing the work done by the doctors, nurses, and staff, and meeting with the residents who used the center. "What impressed him most," wrote Kennedy biographer Adam Clymer, "was seeing women in the waiting room in rocking chairs, where they could look after their children or nurse their babies. He thought that recognized the patient's dignity." Following his three-hour tour of Columbia Point, Kennedy vowed to fight for the community health centers, and, at Geiger's suggestion, drafted an amendment creating an Office of Health Affairs within OEO, providing $100 million to create fifty additional community health centers. "What happened after Kennedy's visit could not happen today," argued Sargent Shriver's biographer Scott Stossel. "It probably could not have happened in any year after 1966. But Democrats still had overwhelming control of both houses of Congress. The budget deficit was . . . not a big worry. Most of all, the New Deal idea that government could solve problems had been revived. So within a couple of months, Kennedy got money for a program of community health centers though Congress." Although the funding was reduced to $50 million in committee, the future of the community health center program was secure.[13]

With financial stability, and the early success of Columbia Point, the future of the Southern health center project was more secure by the beginning of 1966. But as they headed south to select a location for their rural community health center, Geiger and Gibson knew that establishing Columbia Point's sister site was not going to be as quick or as easy. The two envisioned creating a much more comprehensive health center than what was outlined in the OEO guidelines for community health centers—they envisioned approaching health care as a partnership between the poor and the professionals. Their goal was not simply to provide medical care to those in need, but to directly address the social and economic determinates of health. As Geiger told the American Public Health Association in 1966:

We have come to recognize more clearly that we are dealing with a poverty syndrome, a cluster of associated factors: high morbidity, high mortality and low

---

[12] Levitan, "Healing the Poor in their Back Yard," 54.

[13] Levitan, "Healing the Poor in their Back Yard," 54; Clymer, *Edward Kennedy*, 83; Stossel, *Sarge*, 444–46.

utilization of health services; low income; unemployment and unemployability; low education and functional illiteracy; family disorganization and high rates of crime, delinquency and other social pathology; markedly restricted mobility; second third-generation dependency, which we had institutionalized by keeping people on public assistance in abject poverty, by attempts at palliation rather than prevention, and by doing things for, rather than with, poor people; social isolation and powerlessness.[14]

* * *

The driving force behind this book is the same person who spearheaded the creation of the Tufts-Delta Health Center, and, in many ways, the community health center movement in the United States, Dr. H. Jack Geiger. Often referred to as the "father of community health," Geiger's distinguished career includes faculty positons at Harvard University, Tufts University, the State University of New York at Stony Brook, and the City University of New York Medical School, where he founded the Department of Community Health and Social Medicine. He is a founding member of both Physicians for Human Rights and Physicians for Social Responsibility, winning Nobel Prizes with both organizations. Jack Geiger has been awarded nearly every honor possible in his six decades of practicing medicine, but he views the founding of a health center in a poor Mississippi Delta town as one of his most important achievements, and has tried for the past twenty years to have this story told. This book is the culmination of that long effort.

Born in New York City in 1926, Geiger completed medical school after a stint in the Merchant Marine during the Second World War and a brief career as a journalist. While studying at Cleveland's Case Western Reserve Medical School, he became interested in what are now called the "social determinants of health"—how education, poverty, environment, nutrition, and other factors all affect one's health. Geiger was awarded a Rockefeller Foundation fellowship to study the community health centers established in South African townships by Dr. Sidney Kark. Geiger's five months in South Africa were a transformative experience; he saw in practice how creative approaches to health care—looking beyond the treatment of disease to the social determinants of health—could be put into practice, as even the most impoverished populations were empowered to take control over factors that improved their health.

Returning to the United States, Geiger completed his medical education and eventually joined the faculty at Harvard School of Public Health. At this time, his long-held belief in equal rights convinced him to go south and participate in

---

[14] "Delta Health Center Takes Medics to Cotton Turn Rows," Jackson *Clarion-Ledger* (Nov. 14, 1971).

the burgeoning civil rights movement. There he served as a member of the Medical
Committee for Human Rights (MCHR). As a member of MCHR, Geiger worked
with activists, including Martin Luther King Jr. and John Lewis, during some of the
most notable, and violent, demonstrations in Mississippi and Alabama. Geiger and
other members of the MCHR, including Mississippi physicians Robert Smith and
Aaron Shirley, were horrified by the health conditions that they found poor blacks
living in as they followed the civil rights activists throughout the South. Believing
that civil rights for blacks would mean little if health conditions did not improve,
the Medical Committee for Human Rights established the small Mileston Clinic
in Holmes County, Mississippi, one of the poorest counties in the poorest state in
the nation. Beset by financial difficulties, the Mileston Clinic survived less than
two years, but it provided the impetus for Geiger and the MCHR to look for a more
permanent solution to the health crisis in the black South.

Inspired by his work in South Africa with Sidney Kark, Geiger proposed that
a similar community health center model could be established for America's impoverished populations. Working with other members of the MCHR, especially
Dr. Count Gibson of Tufts University Medical School, in 1965 Geiger received a
grant from the new Office of Economic Opportunity to create two demonstration
community health centers, one in the urban North and one in the rural South, as
part of President Lyndon Johnson's War on Poverty. After the nation's first community health center at Columbia Point in Boston was opened in December of 1965,
Geiger selected Mound Bayou, Mississippi, an all-black town deep in the cotton-
rich Delta region, home to some of the poorest people in the nation, as home for
the Southern health center. The Tufts–Delta Health Center began programs the
following year and opened its first permanent facility in 1967. It was an experiment
not only in community health, but in empowering poor people to take more control
of their lives and the circumstances that affected them. A direct outgrowth of the
civil rights movement and a product of the War on Poverty, the Tufts–Delta Health
Center focused not just on delivering health care services, such as immunizations,
check-ups, and medicines, but on aggressively and creatively working to improve the
"social determinants of health" in Bolivar County, Mississippi, through programs
on education, nutrition, and the environment. As it celebrates a half-century of providing care for the region's poor, the Tufts–Delta Health Center (now the Delta
Health Center, Inc.) was the forerunner of more than 1,300 community health centers now operating in the United States and its territories, providing care to over 23
million people annually.

Without intervention, the poor get sicker and the sick get poorer.

—DR. H. JACK GEIGER

I

From South Africa to Mississippi

THE DELTA REGION engulfs the western half of the state of Mississippi, an alluvial plain running 200 miles from Memphis, Tennessee, south to Vicksburg, Mississippi, and stretching approximately seventy miles to the east, encompassing an area of about 7,100 square miles. For centuries it was dense wilderness, regularly flooded by the great river, inhabited only by all manner of wild beasts and a small number of mound-building Native Americans. Starting with Hernando DeSoto, it was claimed at one time or another by all the great colonial powers, but until the nineteenth century it did not see any significant white settlement into its subtropical climate. It was then that the Delta soil, "very dark brown, creamy and sweet smelling, without substrata of rock or shale," according to the planter and author William Alexander Percy, gave rise to a cotton empire built on the backs of slaves, who made up over half of the state's population, and over 80 percent of many Delta counties, at the start of the Civil War. By the time of the war it was some of the most valuable land on earth, and home to some of the nation's wealthiest families, who built the plantation estates that still resonate with most outsiders as the iconic images of the region.[1]

---

[1] James C. Cobb, *The Most Southern Place on Earth* (New York: Oxford University Press), 3, 5–6; William Alexander Percy, *Lanterns on the Levee: Recollections of a Planter's Son* (Alfred A. Knopf, 1941; rpr., LSU press, 1994), 3.

The demise of slavery did not mean the end of King Cotton, and sharecropping emerged as the dominant labor system in the Mississippi Delta, dominated by the freedmen and their descendants. It was an inherently exploitative system, providing plantation owners a control of their labor force that rivaled prewar bondage—and in many ways proved to be much more lucrative to the landowners than slavery had been. Former bondsmen and their families, denied land of their own but refusing to work "like slaves" in the gang-labor system of the past, negotiated with plantation owners—many their former masters—for plots of land that they could work as free men, as if on their own family farm. Landowners initially balked, most preferring to hire former slaves as wage laborers, as a tenant system would produce smaller yields and deprive them of the oversight of their workers to which they were accustomed. The land, however, was only valuable if there were laborers to work it, and within a decade after the end of the war, most plantations had become subdivided into forty- and fifty-acre plots, with small family cabins on them, worked by the former slaves.

In return for their housing and labor, the sharecroppers received a portion—a "share"—of the crop that they had worked at harvest time, usually half, in lieu of rent, but contracts between the tenant and the landowner were negotiated annually. In theory, it was a cooperative arrangement—if the cropper did well and produced a high yield, both he and the landowner profited; if it was a bad year, wracked by flood or drought, both men suffered together. In reality, however, the tally sheets were stacked heavily in the landowner's favor, good years or bad. As the cropper was paid only at harvest time, he survived through the year on credit from the plantation store, where he purchased food for his family, feed for his animals, and sometimes even clothes and tools. If a doctor needed to be called to tend to one of the tenants, his bill would be covered by the plantation owner and added to the yearly bill. Because both the land and the crop were the property of the plantation owner, croppers usually had no say in what was planted, and were rarely allotted any land to grow any food or keep any livestock to feed themselves and their families. The sharecroppers, therefore, lived off credit at the plantation store until the harvest, when, after selling their share (usually through their landowner, who extracted a fee), they settled their tab. More often than not, even in a good year, they found that their yearly earnings were not enough to cover their yearly expenses at the store, especially after the interest was calculated by the landowner. The debt they incurred then tied them to the landowner, who was usually more than willing to have them repeat the cycle again the following year.

By the early twentieth century, stores were often the most profitable enterprises on many plantations, surpassing the value of the actual crops produced. The stores were also the main way to control and maintain a plantation's labor force, turning the sharecroppers into "debt peons," obligated to work the planter's land until their debt was paid. As anyone who has read Faulkner knows, sharecropping not only affected African Americans in the South, but many poor whites as well. Indeed, by the turn of the twentieth century, many small landowners in the South, black and white, had been reduced to tenancy because of their debts to large landowners who acted as furnishing merchants to not only their tenants, but to small farmers in their immediate area. Sharecropping, however, was especially exploitive of African Americans in the Jim Crow South because of their lack of legal recourse against landowners who cheated them on the "figurin'" of yearly accounts, and the use of terror to maintain a docile workforce. The sharecropping economy also contributed directly to the lack of educational opportunities for African Americans in the South as a whole, and Mississippi in particular, as wealthy landowners used their influence to maintain black schools that were not only academically inferior (often to make sure no black child on the plantation could learn how to calculate interest), and to guarantee that schools were closed during the important chopping and harvesting seasons.

Sharecropping began to erode in the 1930s and 1940s, as the Agricultural Adjustment Act (and later the Soil Conservation and Domestic Allotment Act) provided landowners federal subsidies to plow under some of their crops, and leave other fields fallow. Many Southern planters who previously had refused to mechanize their farms now used their federal monies to purchase tractors and mechanical cotton pickers, reducing the need for large numbers of farm laborers. The advent of chemical herbicides, insecticides, and fertilizers further reduced the need for manpower on Southern plantations, and, by the dawn of the 1960s, plantations that used to house five or six families to work the land could be run by two or three hired hands. Some landowners allowed the tenants to remain in their shacks on the plantation, follow the mechanical pickers and collect any stray bits of cotton, and even grow small gardens to support themselves, but others evicted their tenants and burned the shacks to the ground. As one landowner told the *Boston Globe*, "I don't want the niggers on my place, they don't work and I don't take care of them. Oh, I've been letting a few stay on because if I kick them out they'll have no place to go, but that ain't going to last forever."[2]

As the sharecropping system began to die out, many black Southerners fled for jobs in the urban North and West; those who were left in the rural South faced not only unemployment, but a tremendous lack of opportunity to improve their lot in life, due to poverty, lack of education, and systemic racism. One of the

---

[2] John Hatch Collection (private, in possession of the author; hereafter *JHC*); Cynthia Kelly, "Health Care in the Mississippi Delta." *American Journal of Nursing* Vol. 69, No. 4 (April 1969): 758–63; "Tufts Plan: Negroes' Only Ray of Hope," *Boston Globe*, July 16, 1967.

major handicaps that black Southerners faced was the lack of access to medical care; the conditions that so horrified the physicians of the Medical Committee for Human Rights during Freedom Summer were all too common in the rural South. Throughout the region, but especially in the "Black Belt" of Alabama, Mississippi, and Louisiana, rural blacks lacked access to healthcare facilities and providers, and/ or the means to pay for care. Black physicians were rare, and often did not have hospital access, and many white physicians refused to treat black patients at all, or provided Jim Crow care. As one Delta resident recalled, "Most of those doctors made black people use the back door and wait in separate rooms or halls, and they expected you to tell them what was wrong. They seldom examined you, let alone ask you to undress." Another remembered, "Most often I sits on one side of the office and he sits on the other asking questions. There ain't no listening or thumping or looking in the mouth like white folks get." As one civil rights leader commented: "The docs here ain't partial to laying on hands when it comes to treating the colored."[3]

Most physicians—black and white—demanded payment at the time of service. And, in an era before laws mandating emergency treatment regardless of a patient's ability to pay, black patients, even in critical-care situations, were regularly denied access to hospital care, some even dying on hospital steps. One white Mississippi doctor was clear on his attitude toward indigent patients, telling the *Boston Globe*, "If there is a nigger in my waiting room who doesn't have $3 in cash, he can sit there and die. I don't treat niggers without money." Most of the few black physicians in the state, not wanting—or able—to be burdened with only an impoverished clientele, took a similar attitude. "No money, no medicine, it is as simple as that," stated one black physician. "Why, if I was giving away my service, I'd have 'em lined up clear to the Mississippi River." Those unable to pay a private physician often relied on public health clinics open to blacks, which were run by both the state and local governments, but they often provided inadequate or limited treatment, because their major function was providing immunizations, not treating illness. As a result of poor health conditions, in 1960 the black infant mortality rate in Mississippi was 54.4 deaths per 1,000 live births, more than twice the rate for whites, and 5 percent higher than the national black infant mortality rate. In some of Mississippi's Delta counties, black infant mortality rates were greater than 60 per 1,000 live births.[4]

Mississippi's Delta region was one of the areas highlighted by President Lyndon Johnson when he was trying to rally support for the War on Poverty, and it was there that the team from Tufts sought to construct its southern health center. Jack

---

[3] Lefkowitz, *Community Health Centers*, 30; "Sit and Die for Lack of $3," *Boston Globe*, July 17, 1967.

[4] Dittmer, *The Good Doctors*, 81; "Sit and Die for Lack of $3," *Boston Globe*, July 17, 1967; Lefkowitz, *Community Health Centers*, 35–36.

Geiger saw Mississippi as the best location for a demonstration site, because, he said, "I knew if we went to Georgia people would think of Atlanta and think it was better than it really was, but if we went to Mississippi, people would assume it was worse than it really was."[5] By the mid-1960s, however, in the wake of the civil rights movement, Mississippi's white leaders were hostile to any form of federal intervention, including War on Poverty programs. The instituting of Head Start in Mississippi in 1965 had caused a firestorm, with both Mississippi senators James Eastland and John Stennis attacking the program as being tied to both Communists and civil rights groups, and fighting to have the program defunded in the state, while publicly opposing all other Office of Economic Opportunity (OEO) initiatives.[6]

Despite knowing that their program would arouse white hostility in the state, Geiger and Gibson were committed to establishing their center in Mississippi, and began scouting locations for the site in late-1965. As word got out that an OEO-funded health center was being planned for rural Mississippi, local opposition erupted. As Geiger and Gibson reviewed potential sites throughout Mississippi, they met with local physicians, health officers, and hospital administrators who condemned the project as "socialized medicine," and vowed that they would provide no assistance for it. Shockingly, Mississippi's white medical professionals emphasized that such a health center was not even necessary because of the high quality of care that Mississippi's poor already received. Dr. Everett H. Crawford of Tylertown, the state medical association president, said he was "shocked to learn the federal government is seriously considering employing Tufts Medical School to provide comprehensive health services in Mississippi," given that the state medical association saw "no demonstrable reason or necessity for the federal government superimposing a foreign pattern of medical care on the State of Mississippi, [as] our state has a long and honorable history of achievement in public and private medicine which is second to none."[7]

Although Geiger and Gibson would have welcomed support from state politicians and the local white medical establishment, they neither expected nor needed

[5] Sobelson, "Participation, Power, and Place," 44–45.

[6] Chris Meyers Asch, *The Senator and the Sharecropper: The Freedom Struggles of James O. Eastland & Fannie Lou Hamer* (New York and London: The New Press, 2008), 243–44; Michelle Gillette, *Launching the War on Poverty: An Oral History* (New York: Oxford University Press, 2010), 318.

[7] Greta DeJong, "Plantation Politics: The Tufts–Delta Health Center and Interracial Class Conflict in Mississippi, 1965–1972," in Annelise Orleck and Lisa Gayle Hazirjian (Eds.), *The War on Poverty: A New Grassroots History* (Athens: University of Georgia Press, 2011): 256–279; Associated Press Press Release, November 29, 1965, in Series 1, Subseries 1, Box 2, Folder 17, Delta Health Center Records, 1956–1992, Collection 4613, Southern Historical Collection, Wilson Library, University of North Carolina–Chapel Hill (Hereafter *DHC*); "Medical Association Head Opposed to Federal Health Unit," *Sunday Republican* (Waterbury, Conn.), Nov. 26, 1965.

it to get their center up and running. And although governors held veto power over most OEO programs in their states, if the grant was made to an institution of higher learning, then the governor could not veto it. This provision made Tufts's involvement with the health center critical, because it protected the program's funding from a hostile Mississippi government. Southern delegations in Congress, which had fought hard for a governor's veto power over OEO programs, had agreed to this provision with the belief that it would help channel OEO funds to their state universities, and away from local Community Action Programs, which they feared would empower poor and minority communities. They had not considered, however, that an academic institution, like Tufts, might sponsor an OEO program in another state, making it veto-proof from the Mississippi governor. "Tufts was an institution of higher learning; therefore, there was nothing the Mississippi Governor or legislature could do to block it," recalled Geiger. Tufts did not need the approval or support of the local officials, only that they "offer neutrality or toleration" toward the center. Geiger's fear, however, was that too much opposition from Mississippi officials could cause Shriver to kill the program out of political considerations.[8]

The site for the health center soon narrowed to two of Mississippi's Delta counties, Panola and Bolivar, but Geiger already was convinced of the site in Bolivar County when he had visited the town of Mound Bayou in late-1965. Situated in the northeastern part of the county, deep in the Delta, about twenty miles from the Mississippi River, Mound Bayou was an all-black town founded in 1887 by Isaiah T. Montgomery, a former slave of Joseph E. Davis, the brother of the Confederate president Jefferson Davis. Montgomery and his followers sought to create an all-black utopia in the post-Reconstruction South, developing a timber business and growing cotton. By the early twentieth century Mound Bayou stood as beacon of black success in the midst of Jim Crow oppression, with a thriving economy that included a bank, a newspaper, a sawmill, a cotton-oil plant, and a downtown district with stores and churches.[9] In 1942, the Taborian Hospital was opened in the town, owned and run by an African-American fraternal organization, the Knights and Daughters of Tabor. By the time that Geiger and his colleagues were looking for a site to host their health center, however, Mound Bayou had fallen on hard times as the mechanization of the cotton industry resulted in massive black unemployment and outmigration. There were now two small hospitals in the town—the result of a schism in the fraternal order—but both were in desperate straits, in need of financial and professional improvements. Despite these problems, the prospect

---

[8] Gillette, *Launching the War on Poverty*, 319; Sobelson, "Participation, Power, and Place," 72–73.

[9] John C. Willis, *Forgotten Time: The Yazoo–Mississippi Delta After the Civil War* (Charlottesville and London: University Press of Virginia, 2000): 71–73.

of having access to black-run hospitals in a black-run town in the middle of a des-perately poor area in need of help, made Mound Bayou seem to Geiger to be the perfect fit for the location of the new health center.[10]

In order to keep his opposition off-balance, however, Geiger continued to promote the possibility of alternate sites, especially that of Batesville in Panola County, which he knew was less palatable than Mound Bayou to most local white physicians and politicians. Geiger conspicuously visited Batesville to look at potential sites that could be renovated for a health center building, and while at the 1965 annual meeting of the American Medical Association, he and Count Gibson arranged a meeting with the officers of the (all-white) Mississippi Medical Association. At this meeting, which Geiger described as "cordial and professional in tone," Geiger and Gibson presented the case for the health center based on the state's own black morbidity and mortal-ity data, and the near total lack of access to medical care for impoverished black resi-dents. The Mississippi medical leaders then presented their argument that interven-tion was unnecessary. After about an hour of discussion centered on Batesville, Geiger said the only other place they had even considered for a location was the all-black town of Mound Bayou. "The response was instantaneous," Geiger remembered. The Mississippi physicians said they still opposed the project, but if Tufts insisted on going ahead, Mound Bayou was probably the one place in which it could probably be done without much opposition. As Geiger later recalled, "We thus were sanctioned, at this level at least, to go ahead in the place we had really intended all along."[11]

At the same time, Geiger also began to cultivate relationships with some of the black leadership in Mound Bayou, most notably Kemper Smith, the son of Sir P. M. Smith, the founder of the Knights and Daughters of Tabor, which owned one of the hospitals and still held considerable sway with the black community in Bolivar County. Geiger also believed that he was making progress in getting at least the tacit support of some local white officials, including Archie Gray, the direc-tor of the State Board of Health, and Dr. R. T. Hollingsworth, who practiced at Shelby Hospital in Bolivar County. On March 1, 1966, Geiger informed the OEO that Mound Bayou was the choice for the southern health center site. Following the announcement of the center's location, however, vocal opposition to the proj-ect increased. Hollingsworth and Gray changed their tune and came out publicly against the center after Governor Paul Johnson wrote to both Sargent Shriver and Tufts University President Nils Wessell to demand that the center not be located in Mississippi, arguing that the State Board of Health, the Mississippi Medical

---

[10] Lefkowitz, *Community Health Centers*, 37; Thomas J. Ward Jr., *Black Physicians in the Jim Crow South* (Fayetteville: University of Arkansas Press, 2003): 163.

[11] Geiger notes, Jack Geiger Collection (private, in the possession of the author; hereafter *JGC*).

Association, and the Mississippi Association of Hospital Administrators all opposed the project. The health center proposal also was attacked by both politicians
and the local press as being little more than a cover for civil rights groups. Following
this barrage of opposition, on March 31 Geiger received a letter from OEO suspend-
ing the Bolivar County project.[12]

On April 13, in an attempt to both rally support for, and diffuse suspicions about
the center, Geiger spoke to the physicians of the Delta Medical Society. He not
only had to contend with their fears that a federally-funded health center would
harm them economically by cutting into their patient base, but also deal with the
tremendous distrust that this overwhelmingly white organization had developed
during the civil rights movement of outsiders and the federal government coming
into Mississippi to do anything for African Americans. On this last account, Jack
Geiger could probably have not been a worse advocate for the center. A Northern
Jew who was with Dr. King in Selma, he was everything that this group feared.
The secretary of the Delta Medical Society, Dr. Howard Nelson, told the OEO that
Geiger "lost the fight" with the audience "when he admitted that he had been involved in the civil rights movement in Mississippi in the past and that the people in
the project would continue to be concerned about civil rights." Other participants
at the meeting were more diplomatic, but just as unenthusiastic, about the center as
Dr. Nelson, stating that they were "suspicious about the project," which they "fear
will interfere with progress in other anti-poverty programs," and that "Tufts needs
to describe carefully the scope and details of its proposed work."[13]

At the end of the meeting the physicians voted 50–1 against the proposed health
center. (The one vote in support of the plan was the lone black physician in attendance, who, of all the physicians present, probably faced the greatest threat to his
economic livelihood if the center was built.) Despite this result, Geiger was thrilled,
because almost thirty members abstained from the vote, indicating to Geiger that
they understood the need for the center and were willing to support his efforts, as
long as their support was not on the public record. His assessment was confirmed
that evening when at a dinner sponsored by the medical society a number of the
physicians quietly pulled him aside and told him, "You go ahead and do that. That's
a good thing you want to do." Geiger then realized that "that there was a substantial
reservoir of latent support that people were not about to articulate publicly because
of the social costs to them, but that it was there."[14]

---

[12] DeJong, "Plantation Politics," 256–79; Geiger notes, *JGC*.

[13] Memo from Ted Berry to Sargent Shriver, 4/14/66, *JGC*.

[14] Sobelson, "Participation, Power, and Place," 74–75; Interview with Jack Geiger by Robert Korstad and Neil
Boothby.

Finding that the OEO report on the meeting focused on the vote in opposition to the health center, on May 26 Geiger flew to Washington, unannounced, along with the vice president of Tufts, to pitch their case to Shriver. After a contentious situation, where the men refused to leave Shriver's office until they met with the director (an OEO "sit-in," as Geiger later referred to it), they held a five-hour meeting with Shriver's deputy, Dr. Julius Richmond, the director of Head Start. Arguing that refusing Tufts's application to open the Mississippi Health Center would send a signal to all other universities not to sponsor or cooperate with OEO projects, an agreement eventually was brokered, and Shriver approved the Mound Bayou site.[15]

* * *

H. Jack Geiger, the son of a physician father and microbiologist mother, had grown up on the Upper West Side of Manhattan, "about as far away from a cotton field as you can get," he later remembered with a laugh. A tremendously gifted student, Geiger graduated from high school at age fourteen, but was constantly in conflict with his parents. Befriended by the noted African-American actor Canada Lee after meeting him following a performance of the stage adaptation of *Native Son*, Geiger began to spend time at the actor's home, even moving in for a while. Lee was a member of the black intelligentsia of the 1930s and 1940s, and at Lee's home Geiger came into contact with the black artistic and political elite—including Duke Ellington, Paul Robeson, Langston Hughes, Richard Wright, and Adam Clayton Powell—where his passion for racial justice was inspired. With financial assistance from Lee, Geiger matriculated at the University of Wisconsin and majored in journalism. At Wisconsin he continued to cultivate his interest in civil rights, emerging as an activist against segregated campus housing and founding one of the nation's earliest chapters of the Congress of Racial Equality (CORE).[16]

During World War II, Geiger left Wisconsin and enlisted in the Merchant Marine, the only branch of the service that was not racially segregated at that time. He served on the *SS Booker T. Washington*, the only ship in the merchant fleet with a black captain and an integrated crew of officers. Following his three years of service, Geiger entered the University of Chicago as a premed student and continued his involvement in civil rights activities, serving as the civil liberties chairman of the American Veterans Committee, and engaging in protests to integrate Grant Park and the Avalon Ballroom. He raised awareness of the exclusion of blacks at the University of Chicago's medical school and hospitals, leading a long-running campaign against racial discrimination at the university, including a day-long protest strike attended by more than one thousand students and faculty. His civil rights

---

[15] Geiger notes, *JGC*; Interview with Jack Geiger by Robert Korstad and Neil Boothby.
[16] Dittmer, *The Good Doctors*, 63–65; Interview with Jack Geiger by Robert Korstad and Neil Boothby.

activities did not go unnoticed, and when he applied to medical school he found that he had been blackballed by the American Medical Association, whose vice president had sent a letter to the dean of every U.S. medical school, calling attention to Geiger's "extra-curricular activities." Denied admission to medical school, Geiger took a job as the science editor for the International News Service, where he covered medicine for the next four years. Eventually, in 1954, at age twenty-nine, he was admitted to Western Reserve (now Case Western) Medical School in Cleveland, Ohio, where he began to combine his twin passions of medicine and civil rights advocacy.[17]

During his second year at Western Reserve, Geiger had an epiphany while standing on the medical school steps. "You could see the teaching hospital, beyond which you could see the city of Cleveland," he recalled. "And it occurred to me that in Cleveland, who got sick, and who didn't, and what happened to them and their interactions were not just biological phenomena; they were social, economic, political, and racial phenomena." Though he thought he had discovered this connection between health and living conditions, he soon found out that "social medicine" had been examined by the British and Germans more than a century before. Inspired by this connection, he sought to explore the field more deeply and applied to the Rockefeller Foundation for a grant to pursue studies in international health. He received a five-month fellowship to study community-oriented primary care at community health centers in both urban and rural South African townships, which were at that time flourishing with aid from the Rockefeller Foundation. It would be in South Africa that the genesis of the Tufts–Delta Health Center emerged.[18]

In South Africa, Geiger worked under the direction of Drs. Sidney and Emily Kark, who had pioneered the development of community health centers in some of the poorest black townships of South Africa. Born in Johannesburg in 1911, Sidney Kark graduated from Witwatersrand University Medical School (South Africa) in 1936. While at Witwatersrand he met his future wife, Emily Jaspan, and, even before they had graduated from medical school, the two began to work toward improving the lives of South Africa's black majority, founding the Society for the Study of Medical Conditions among the Bantu, which initiated health surveys of black children in South Africa. These surveys found widespread malnutrition among black children, resulting in all types of disease and appalling infant mortality. In 1940, the two physicians, now husband and wife, were appointed by the government health

---

[17] Dittmer, *The Good Doctors*, 63–65; Interview with Jack Geiger by Robert Korstad and Neil Boothby; Richard Hall, "A Stir of Hope in Mound Bayou," *LIFE* (March 28, 1969): 67–79; Geiger notes, *JGC*.

[18] Dittmer, *The Good Doctors*, 63–65; Interview with Jack Geiger by Robert Korstad and Neil Boothby; Sobelson, "Participation, Power and Place," 37–38.

department to create an experimental health unit at Pholela, a rural African "tribal reserve" in Natal province. At Pholela they developed the program of "community-oriented primary care" for which they later became famous, and which would eventually have a great impact on the Tufts–Delta Health Center in Mississippi. Their program focused not just on health care delivery to individuals, but on the health of the entire community—in essence, everyone in the community was considered a patient. Clinical services were combined with traditional public health care along with educational, environmental, and nutrition programs. The program also sought to empower the community to improve its own health. In doing so, it developed innovative community outreach programs, as the Karks recruited and trained locals as health workers, and even worked with the community's traditional healers. As Sidney Kark remarked, "Understanding the people's beliefs, customs, and life style was an important aspect in their training."[19]

The community health center at Pholela proved to be such a success that, in 1946, the Karks moved to Durban, where Sidney directed the newly created Institute of Family and Community Health (IFCH). The mission of the IFCH was to train personnel for a network of health centers based on the Pholela model, and by the mid-1950s South Africa had established forty such centers across the nation in black, Indian, and poor white communities. The entire network of community health centers was sponsored by the University of Natal, South Africa's only medical school for nonwhites, where Sidney Kark had established a Department of Community Medicine. The clinics were open to anyone, sick or well, regardless of ability to pay. In an attempt to combine both preventive and curative care, programs conducted by the centers ranged from traditional health services like immunizations and epidemic disease control, to more innovative programs in nutrition, housing, and environmental health. Community health nurses left the confines of the centers and visited homes and schools. Epidemiological surveys of the communities were conducted to ascertain best what the most pressing health needs were, as were health surveys of all schoolchildren in the center's area. Educational programs were instituted on topics as varied as diet, insect control, latrines, and gardening.[20]

---

[19] Sidney and Emily Kark, *Promoting Community Health: From Pholela to Jerusalem* (Johannesburg, South Africa: Witwatersrand University Press, 1999), *vi–vii*, 5–6, 25; Theodore Brown and Elizabeth Fee, "Sidney Kark and John Cassel: Social Medicine Pioneers and South African Emigrés," *American Journal of Public Health* (November 2002) 92 (11): 1744–45; Lefkowitz, *Community Health Centers*, 6–7.

[20] H. Jack Geiger, "The First Community Health Centers," 313–14; Brown and Fee, "Sidney Kark and John Cassel," 1744–45; Kark and Kark, *Promoting Community Health*, 28–30; "Community Health: A Model for the World," in *Against the Odds: Making a Difference in Global Health*, U.S. National Library of Medicine (http://apps.nlm.nih.gov/againsttheodds/exhibit/community_health/model_world.cfm)

Despite their success, the Karks faced tremendous opposition to their community-oriented primary care, not only from white government officials, but from local black leaders as well. Sidney Kark found that, "The tribal leaders, fearing the imposition by officialdom of a new, unwanted and unrequested government institution in their midst, ... [appealed] to have the health center removed," while "some of the local elders attempted to arouse the people against the acceptance of our health team and the services we proposed to introduce." He found, therefore, that one of the first, and most difficult, hurdles he had to overcome was convincing the population he sought to serve that he could be trusted and that they should indeed welcome his program. Geiger later would encounter much the same reception from some local black leaders in Mississippi. "It was clear that we would have to find acceptance in the community," recalled Kark, "and to do so we would have to hold numerous discussions with community leaders and with the local Pholela authorities." In addition to local black opposition, as the Apartheid regime hardened in the 1950s, it, too, became very critical of the community health centers in general, and Sidney Kark in particular. He was placed under surveillance, regularly harassed by the government, and even investigated for alleged communist sympathies, not because of any links with communist organizations, but because of the health center's practice of distributing free milk to malnourished children.[21]

Geiger apprenticed under Karks for five months in 1957 at both the original community health center in rural Pholela and at an urban Zulu housing project, Lamontville, in Durban. Many of the ideas for the Tufts–Delta Health Center— from university sponsorship of the center to the environmental and nutrition programs it provided—originated from his experiences in South Africa. At both Pholela and Lamontville, Geiger recalled, "I would examine patients in a consulting room that had plastered on the walls graphs and histograms of the infant mortality rate by race and section of the community. The typhoid rate, the immunization rates, and all kinds of pertinent epidemiologic and demographic information." He fully understood then that, "One could not treat the individual patient without thinking about the community." When he returned to the United States, he wrote a thesis, which was required for his medical degree at Western Reserve, entitled "Family Health in Three Cultures: Implications for Medical Education," which contrasted his work at Lamontville and Pholela with the outpatient departments at Western Reserve's teaching hospitals. He concluded his thesis with the recommendation that an American medical school start a community health center. "It

---

[21] Kark and Kark, *Promoting Community Health, xiii,* 23–24; "Community Health: A Model for the World."

was the first proposal that I know of for what became community health centers in this country," recalled Geiger.[22]

Not long after Geiger left Pholela and Lamontville, the political climate in South Africa became too oppressive for the Karks, and they (along with a number of their colleagues at the IFCH), left South Africa. The Karks spent a year in the University of North Carolina's School of Public Health, and in 1959 went to Jerusalem as part of a three-year World Health Organization–Israel project to establish a Department of Social Medicine at the Hebrew University Hadassah Medical School. Sidney Kark became professor and head of the Department of Social Medicine there, where he served until his retirement in 1980; he died in 1998.[23]

Because of his experience in South Africa, Geiger realized that merely establishing a medical clinic in the Mississippi Delta would amount to little more than a bandage on the health problems of its impoverished residents. Instead, what was needed was a comprehensive, community-based approach to solving the health problems of the Delta, as had been done in South Africa. Therefore, before there would be any vaccinations given or babies delivered, there had to be a thorough evaluation of the situation in the Delta, and, as Kark had learned in South Africa, the cultivation of a positive relationship with the local community. To accomplish this task he hired John Hatch, a social worker and community organizer with the Boston Housing Authority. Hatch had just been appointed to the Tufts faculty to help develop the new health center at Columbia Point when he met Count Gibson. "Count Gibson influenced my thinking of the role of social action and health," Hatch remembered. "I was so excited of learning of the intention to develop a model comprehensive health center in the South" that "I left the safety of the Boston Housing Authority to join the team." Even before the location for the southern health center had been settled upon, Geiger tapped Hatch to scout possible locations in Mississippi.[24]

A bear of a man, quiet, with kind eyes and a warm smile, John Hatch presented quite a contrast to the loquacious Geiger. A child of the segregated South, Hatch was born in Kentucky in 1928; his college-educated father was the principal of the local Rosenwald school and pastor of the African Methodist Zion church. "Relative to other African-American families, we were better off," he remembered, but he was still subject to inferior segregated education, "without libraries or laboratories." Nevertheless, he attended the Kentucky State College for Negroes, and planned on a career in the law, eventually becoming the first student enrolled at the temporary

---

[22] Interview with Jack Geiger by Robert Korstad and Neil Boothby.

[23] Brown and Fee, "Sidney Kark and John Cassel," 1744–45.

[24] John Hatch Narrative, *JHC.*

law school for blacks set up in the state to maintain segregation. When the National Association for the Advancement of Colored People (NAACP) succeeded in having such arrangements deemed unconstitutional, he enrolled at the state law school in Lexington, becoming the first black law student at the University of Kentucky. The law school dean, however, required that empty chairs be set up next to him in class in an attempt to provide a modicum of segregation. Unwilling to stand for such humiliation, Hatch left law school after one semester and taught high school in Arkansas before being drafted in 1952.[25]

After serving in the Korean War, Hatch was discharged in 1955, but found that it was now "more difficult to deal with dirty, single-sex toilets, back row seating and discourteous bus agents and drivers than three years earlier." He enrolled in Knoxville College, graduating two years later with a degree in sociology, and then entered the graduate program in community organization at the Atlanta University School of Social Work. In Atlanta he also began to work part-time for the NAACP, doing interviews of potential plaintiffs for the Atlanta school desegregation lawsuit. Graduating with a Master's in Social Work in 1961, he left the South for Boston, taking a position as a community organizer and youth worker in the city's South End. In 1963, married and with a young family, he took a secure, well-paid position with the Boston Housing Authority. "I was . . . the highest ranking black person within the Housing Authority's administrative structure," he recalled. "I really had made it, in that it's a tenured position that you can hold the rest of your life that paid enough to live off of comfortably. A number of people thought I was absolutely insane to leave a job with such great security," he recalled after Geiger and Gibson offered him the position with Tufts. He also questioned whether it would be fair to his wife, a Boston native, and their children, to move from the New England suburbs to the rural South, but the "desire to be socially useful, and the belief that things can be better. . . . That there is a vast reservoir of good and decent people who, given choices, will do things that enhance the quality of their lives and the life of the community," proved too strong of an attraction to keep Hatch in Boston. He agreed to go to Mississippi, where he became an integral part of the health project.[26]

If Jack Geiger was the heart of the Tufts–Delta Health Center, then John Hatch was its soul. While Geiger secured funding and planned the center, Hatch was on the ground in Bolivar County, building relationships and trust among the local black

[25] John Hatch Narrative, *JHC*; George C. Wright, *A History of Blacks in Kentucky, Volume 2: In Pursuit of Equality, 1890–1980* (Frankfort: Kentucky Historical Society, 2001), 178.

[26] John Hatch Narrative, *JHC*; Interview with John Hatch by Robert Korstad and Neil Boothby, May 26, 1992. Southern Rural Poverty Collection (http://dewitt.sanford.duke.edu/wp-content/uploads/2011/09/HATCH1.pdf).

community that Geiger—as a white, urban, Yankee—had no hope of developing, but that were instrumental if the health center was to have any success. Although opposition from white segregationists was expected by the advocates of the health center, suspicion and even outward hostility toward the project from the local black community took many of the project's leaders by surprise. Hatch understood that gaining local black support for the health center was just as essential—and perhaps just as difficult—as diffusing white opposition. "Contact with the community was necessary [for the success of the project]," he recalled. "Most of us had done some reading in community health and were all too familiar with the number of very excellently staffed facilities that fell flat when they attempted to intervene interchanging local practices around various aspects of health care."[27]

Upon arriving in the Mississippi Delta in the fall of 1965, Hatch did not first set to community organizing, as he had been doing in Boston, but instead tried to integrate himself with the local population in the best way he could think of. "I'd not lived in the rural South for over 15 years. I thought it useful to reorient myself to patterns of interactions and thought, and in a rural farm worker environment," Hatch recalled, so he lived with sharecropping families in plantation shacks and joined cotton-picking crews in the Delta. "After picking for half a day, my hands bleeding, back aching, and vision blurred, I picked 80 pounds of cotton. This woman, twice my age, had picked 150 pounds and seemed as fresh as when she began at 7:30 a.m." Hatch was out of touch for so long, that back in Boston Geiger began to worry about his safety, but Hatch's experiment was successful in that he had abundant time to speak with the farm workers about their economic and health situations, even if they often questioned exactly why he was there. "They were curious about me," he remembered. "Most doubted I came from Boston to Mississippi to learn about social change. Several thought [I was] running from personal trouble up north and needed a place to hide."[28]

Along with working in the cotton fields, Hatch spent several months living with poor black residents of the Delta, sharing not only their work, but also their social life, along with their everyday problems. "Experiencing diarrhea in a crowded rural home without toilet facilities is considerably more impressionable than reviewing data on the high rate of intestinal disorder, its probable cause, and the statistical fact that 90 percent of the housing is dilapidated and without plumbing," he later remarked in a paper on his experiences. What he learned was that not only was there a great need for improved health care—"we knew that from statistics," he

[27] Interview with John Hatch, Delta Health Center Tapes, Disk 1, Reel 5-2.
[28] John Hatch Narrative, *JHC*.

recalled—but improvement in how people coped with the everyday problems they faced, as well as how they dealt with crises and emergencies. "Knowledge of how sick people were tended to, how the community reached out to isolated elderly and so forth was really critical as we began to assess intervention strategies," he remembered as some of the most valuable lessons of that time living with the people of the Mississippi Delta.[29]

As Hatch scouted the area, and as plans moved forward for the health center, the expected resistance and opposition from the local white population to a health center funded by the federal government and staffed with Yankee physicians from a medical school in Boston—perhaps no combination of factors could have been more abhorrent to a white Mississippian in the mid-1960s—continued to mount, from local physicians all the way up to the governor. Arguments against the center ranged from its lack of support from the local medical societies and fears that it would put local physicians out of business, to assertions that black residents of the Delta already received adequate health care and the clinic was therefore not necessary. Dr. A. L. Gray, the head of Mississippi's Department of Public Health, summed up the main argument of the state's opposition to the center in a 1966 interview: "We're opposed to the idea of the center, of course. We feel that any work like that should come to recognize the established state or local agencies. All this is from outside, with no state or local sanction of any kind that I know about." When the Tufts group cited evidence of the numerous health deficiencies in the region, including some of the highest black infant mortality rates in the nation—the Mississippi doctors and politicians then changed their tune, arguing that they, not Tufts, should receive the federal monies to improve health care in the region. As one local white physician argued, "This is not to mean that we're opposed to services for these people need it and should have it. We just think that our health department is well qualified to do that kind of work and should be administering a fund like that."[30]

Although most OEO programs were, indeed, designed to be run by local groups, with maximum feasible participation from the affected communities, to the Tufts team the idea of having local white authorities administer the proposed health center was anathema, given that they believed that it would do absolutely no good to turn over federal funds to precisely the people who, in their view, had neglected black health care for so long. "We . . . kept saying, 'What is the problem with taking

---

[29] John Hatch, "Community Development in a Rural Comprehensive Community Health Program," paper presented at the New York Academy of Medicine annual health conference, April 24, 1970, *JHC*; Interview with John Hatch by Robert Korstad and Neil Boothby.

[30] "Mississippians Protest OEO Plans for Bolivar County Health Center," *Memphis Commercial-Appeal*, February 4, 1966.

care of poor people who are miserably sick and don't have access to health care? How can anybody object to that? It is quite clear that it is not being done with available resources'," Geiger recalled arguing. "To which the best they could say was, 'Well, give the money to us and we'll take care of it'—all of this huge amount of money that was being proposed. We said, obviously, their record wasn't good and there were none of these other elements of community participation."[31]

To charges that they were creating a system of "socialized medicine" that would run local physicians out of business, Geiger countered that the proposed center, while open to all, was designed to serve those individuals and families the traditional "pay-for-service" medical system left behind. "I'm most concerned that we do not create economic competition with physicians in the area or damage their practices, and we would make every effort to see that this does not occur," wrote Geiger to Dr. Robert Hollingsworth of Shelby, Mississippi, "[but] I find it hard to believe the populations with an annual family income of $900 a year or less can contribute significantly to the practice incomes of physicians, or that a county with a physician-to-population ratio of 40 per 100,000 persons—as compared to the national average of 135 per 100,000 persons—cannot use additional medical facilities."[32]

One of the most strenuous points of opposition to the project had nothing to do with health care at all, but with a belief held by many in the white community that the health center (and most OEO programs) were nothing more than a cover for civil rights activities, backed by federal dollars. Geiger and Gibson understood that political action by the health center would jeopardize their project, and assured OEO leadership that they would not engage in partisan action, writing that, "Governor Johnson can be assured that the health center, [as a] university function, will not engage in partisan political activity. Of course, Tufts University is a law abiding institution and Governor Johnson can be further assured a health center will abide by all relevant national, state, and local statutes." They also asserted, however, that "the Tufts program *by its very nature and premises* [was] committed to a concern for human rights, in particular the right to health, and that it believes full participation of Negro citizens and a health program is essential to achieve this goal."[33]

Along with white opposition to the project, a significant—and powerful—segment of the local black population was also very wary of the proposed health center, including: medical practitioners who feared competition; traditional elites who had controlled the Mound Bayou's political and economic life for decades,

---

[31] Interview with H. Jack Geiger by Robert Korstad and Neil Boothby.

[32] Letter from H. Jack Geiger to Dr. Robert Hollingsworth, March 15, 1966, *JGC*.

[33] Letter from Count Gibson and H. Jack Geiger to Julius Richmond, MD, Director of Health Programs, OEO, April 27, 1966, *JGC*.

and feared a (potentially lucrative) operation that was out of their control; and even some black militants opposed to a wealthy "white" institution inundating a famous all-black community to provide services to poor blacks. A great deal of distrust also existed as to the motives of both Tufts and the federal government—why would they want to spend time, money, and energy on poor black people in the Mississippi Delta? What was in it for them? As one black Delta resident recalled, there was some "fear and some concern about why [Tufts would] come down here and give us free healthcare," including rumors that clinic patients might be experimented upon. One report to Tufts President Nils Wessel in early 1966 echoed this sentiment, stating, "[the black people] are quite frank to point out that so much has been promised and so little has been given historically, that they view all offers somewhat wearily." Part of John Hatch's job was, therefore, to try and win over those in the black community who either felt threatened by, or were distrustful of, the prospect of a federally-funded health center in the Mound Bayou. Thanks in great part to Hatch's work on the ground, efforts to mollify black concerns were generally successful. According to Hatch, "our accessibility and willingness to talk probably diffused several potentially explosive situations."[34]

By early 1966, Hatch returned to Boston and the decision was made to locate the health center in the town of Mound Bayou and have it serve the residents of the northern half of Bolivar County. Because of its history, location, facilities, and obvious need, the all-black town of Mound Bayou seemed to be the perfect location. Geiger had certainly thought so when he had visited in 1965, and Hatch's time in the Delta had confirmed many of the advantages that Mound Bayou presented. One advantage that Mound Bayou seemed to provide for the health center was a modicum of protection from white discrimination. Because of the town's history of black prosperity and relative isolation from hostile whites, Geiger believed that Mound Bayou would provide "a degree of shelter from the state and a degree of physical safety for an integrated staff which in other areas might have been considerably more problematic." There were other practical concerns; as Hatch later recalled, "we thought it would be . . . more challenging to find accommodation in the towns that were still under white control and oppression, than in Mount Bayou where we thought there would be relatively easier acceptance."[35] The fact that the town's government, as well as all its municipal facilities, were all black-run—an incredible oddity in 1960s Mississippi—seemed to augur well for locating the center there.

[34] Dittmer, *The Good Doctors*, 230; John Hatch Narrative, *JHC*; Letter from Frank A. Tredinick Jr. to Nils Wessel, March 25, 1966, *JGC*; Sobelson, "Participation, Power, and Place," 62–63.

[35] Interview with H. Jack Geiger by Robert Korstad and Neil Boothby; Interview with John Hatch by Robert Korstad and Neil Boothby.

Another significant attribute that the town had was a long history of providing medical care for African Americans in the Delta. In 1926 Perry M. Smith, a Mississippi school teacher, was elected chief grand mentor of the Mississippi Jurisdiction of the Knights and Daughters of Tabor. When Smith took over the Mississippi arm of the society its membership was floundering. In order to revive the chapter, Smith decided to emulate the success of other African-American fraternal organizations and build a hospital to provide inexpensive health care for the society's members. He first proposed his hospital plan in 1929, but it was rejected by the organization's membership. Undaunted, he continued to press for a society hospital throughout the 1930s, and in 1938 the membership finally consented to raising $100,000 for a facility to be built in Mound Bayou. Funding for the Knights and Daughters of Tabor Hospital was raised primarily from an assessment on the 25,000 members of the society, and on February 1, 1942, the one-story, forty-two-bed Taborian Hospital opened in Mound Bayou.[36]

Taborian Hospital was a boon to blacks in the Mississippi Delta. Drs. W. L. Smith of Clarksville and Phillip M. George of Mound Bayou codirected the facility, and Dr. Theodore Howard was hired as surgeon-in-chief. Howard was a surgeon at Meharry Medical College's Hubbard Hospital in Nashville when he was approached by Smith to be chief surgeon at Taborian. At that time Meharry was the only medical school in the South open to African Americans, and, along with Howard University Medical School in Washington, DC, produced the vast majority of the nation's black physicians. Dr. Howard accepted the position and soon emerged as both the hospital's dominant force, and a leading figure in Mound Bayou, eventually amassing a substantial fortune in both business and medicine. Under his guidance, within four years the facility was expanded to seventy-six beds, and by 1946 the hospital conducted more than 1,200 operations annually in its two operating rooms. Members of the Knights and Daughters of Tabor who paid the annual Hospital Emergency Tax of $2 and the quarterly hospital fee of $.75 (1943 rates) were entitled to up to thirty-one days a year of free hospitalization in Taborian's wards, including all their medical and surgical examinations and treatments. Nonmembers also were admitted to the hospital, but at higher costs. There was tremendous demand for the service that Taborian Hospital provided. Howard

---

[36] Ward Jr., *Black Physicians in the Jim Crow South*, 146–47; David Beito, "Black Fraternal Hospitals of the Mississippi Delta," *The Journal of Southern History*, February 1999): 109–40; *The Taborian Star* (Cary, Mississippi), March 1942; Matthew Walker, "The Affiliation of Taborian Hospital with Meharry Medical College and Development of the OEO Planning Grant," *Meharry Medical College Quarterly Digest* 4 (April 1966): 3; Hodding Carter, "He's Doing Something About the Race Problem," *Saturday Evening Post* (February 23, 1946): 31. For more on the development of the nation's black hospitals, see Vanessa Northington Gamble's *Making a Place for Ourselves* (New York: Oxford University Press, 1995).

told journalist Hodding Carter in 1946 that there was a "long waiting list" of patients wanting to be treated at the hospital, and that "even the demand for private rooms is twenty times the supply." Howard credited Taborian's success to the fact that "Negroes want good care too. These days a good many of them can pay for care. But in too many of Mississippi's too few hospitals Negroes have to bring their own sheets and spoons and someone to give them nursing care. And, in many cases, the accommodations are dirtier than you'd believe."[37]

Mound Bayou also had been the site of a significant public health project that would, in many ways, foreshadow the development of the Tufts–Delta Health Center three decades later. In the summer of 1935, Dr. Dorothy Ferebee of Howard University's School of Medicine began a six-week public health clinic for impoverished African Americans of the Mississippi Delta. Centered at the Saints Industrial School in Holmes County and sponsored by the Alpha Kappa Alpha (AKA) sorority, Dr. Ferebee, her volunteers, and two public health nurses on loan from the county health department, traveled from plantation to plantation, providing immunizations and physical exams for children, and giving demonstrations to adults on sanitation, diet, and preventative health care.[38]

Because of hostility from many plantation owners, the sorority decided to relocate the health clinic to Bolivar County the next year, and from 1936 to 1941 Dr. Ferebee and her team of volunteers descended on Mound Bayou each summer to provide free health care for the area's black residents. The town of Mound Bayou put the project's volunteers up in private homes throughout the city, and the mayor pledged all the support that he could muster to make the program a success for the Delta's black citizens. The initial clinic in 1936 was held at the Mound Bayou schoolhouse, and in its first two days over 500 children and adults were treated. After the inaugural clinic was completed, the project took to the back roads of Bolivar County. The county was broken up into four districts, with thirty-two total clinic sites. Clinics usually were operated in two separate locations on any given day, but sometimes as many as three clinics were held on the same day. In addition to the support of the town of Mound Bayou and the Bolivar County Health Department, local newspapers ran announcements for the clinics, and posters were hung in schools, churches, and stores. For the most part Bolivar County's white population was supportive of

[37] Ward, *Black Physicians in the Jim Crow South*, 146–47; *The Taborian Star* (Cary, Miss.), March 1942, Feb. 1943; Carter, "He's Doing Something About the Race Problem," 31, 64; Herbert M. Morais, Ed., *The History of the Afro-American in Medicine* (Cornwell Heights, Pa.: The Publisher's Agency, 1978), 149–50. For more on Taborian Hospital, see David T. Beito, *From Mutual Aid to the Welfare State* (Chapel Hill, N.C. and London, 2000), 181–203.

[38] Ward, *Black Physicians in the Jim Crow South*, 242–44.

the project, in no small part due to the efforts of the county's health director who was enthusiastic about having the clinics held in his county. The school board gave AKA permission to use the colored schools of the county for the clinics; local newspapers ran announcements for the clinics; posters were hung in schools, churches, and stores; and white landowners made provision for their tenants to attend the programs. The AKA's Mississippi Health Project was suspended during World War II because of gasoline rationing, and then never resumed.[39]

Because of its unique history, Mound Bayou seemed to be the perfect location for the proposed Tufts–Delta Health Center, but problems with locating the center there began to emerge even before the center was even ready to see its first patients. Although the town did rightfully boast a proud racial history that included numerous successful businesses (although most had withered or died by the 1960s), and a legacy of political independence, both of these factors also had created significant class divisions within the town—divisions that would prove to cause significant conflicts with the health center in the future. John Hatch had even been warned by local civil rights leaders that Mound Bayou might not be the optimal place to locate the center. Cleveland, Mississippi's Amzie Moore, a World War II veteran and NAACP organizer, consulted with Hatch during his scouting of locations in the Delta. Moore advised against placing the center in Mound Bayou, and indicated that if it was placed there he would not have anything to do with it. During the movement years, Moore had become frustrated with Mound Bayou's ruling class, whom he believed felt themselves superior to poor blacks in the region, and had not contributed much to the movement because, as Moore stated, "they think they're already free," because they could vote in local elections and controlled the town government.[40]

As Moore predicted, friction with Mound Bayou's ruling elites soon emerged as details of the center became known. As historian Greta DeJong wrote, "Class stratification, exploitation, and the monopolization of political power by the town's wealthiest citizens characterized Mound Bayou. . . . Mound Bayou's black leaders appealed to residents' racial pride and minimize challenges to their dominance." The prospect of a million dollar federal health center in their town, and the jobs it

[39] Ward, *Black Physicians in the Jim Crow South*, 244–48; AKA Sorority, *The 1936 Mississippi Health Project in Bolivar County* (pamphlet), in Folder 4, Box 183–17, Dorothy Ferebee Papers, Howard University, Washington, DC (hereafter *DFP*); Ella Payne Morgan, "A Project Conducted in Mississippi: Alpha Kappa Alpha Sorority Health Project, 1935–1942," Howard University student paper, August 1942, in Folder 6, Box 183–17, *DFP*; Ratliff, "Cotton Field Clinic," *DFP*.

[40] Cobb, *The Most Southern Place on Earth*, 211; Sobelson, "Participation, Power, and Place," 77; Hatch narrative, *JHC*; Interview with H. Jack Geiger by Robert Korstad and Neil Boothby.

would create, all controlled by outsiders—most of them white—was very threatening to those who ran the town.[41]

Another problem was the condition of Mound Bayou's two hospitals, which were both in tremendous disrepair in the 1960s. In 1946, a schism developed among the leaders of the Taborian Hospital, which eventually resulted in the dismissal of Dr. Howard as surgeon-in-chief. Howard, who also ran a private clinic in Mound Bayou (one of the sources of conflict that led to his dismissal from Taborian), responded by rallying supporters and forming a rival fraternal society, the United Order of Friendship, which opened its own smaller hospital in Mound Bayou in 1948 (first known as the Friendship Clinic, and later as the Sara Brown Hospital) and named Howard surgeon-in-chief. By the 1960s, with the collapse of the sharecropping economy and subsequent erosion in the number of those who could pay fraternal hospital insurance, both facilities were struggling financially and unable to maintain their facilities up to acceptable standards. Indeed, if it were not for Mississippi's lax hospital regulation and a desire to maintain segregation, both hospitals already might have been shut down. According to historian David Beito, local white physicians actually campaigned to keep the all-black hospitals open, fearing that if they were closed, the patients they served would put too much pressure on the county's charity care.[42]

For his part, Geiger was horrified by the condition of the two fraternal hospitals. In a 1966 letter he described the hospitals as "physically deteriorating, fiscally unsound . . ., understaffed, and inadequately planned. . . . There is a fundamental absurdity in the situation of two small institutions, neither adequately financed nor physically prepared to carry the burden of in-hospital medical care for the population it serves, standing across the street from one another in direct competition with each other, with two inadequate operating rooms, two inadequate x-ray units, two grossly inadequate laboratories, and so on." Geiger's criticism might be understood as the reaction of someone—coming from Boston—accustomed to the most modern hospital amenities, and not appreciating difficulties faced by small, poor, rural, and segregated facilities. Indeed, Count Gibson tempered his criticism of Mound Bayou's hospitals, stating that "it all depends on . . . perspective. Here were our doctors trained in Northern hospitals coming down to look at this. How many other little rural hospitals, black or white, might not have been that different?" John Hatch's assessment, however, was no better than Geiger's, characterizing Taborian's

---

[41] DeJong, "Plantation Politics," 259, 268.

[42] Beito, "Black Fraternal Hospitals in Mississippi Delta, 1942–1967," 120–21, 128. For more on Dr. Theodore Mason Howard, see David Beito's *Black Maverick: T.R.M. Howard's Fight for Civil Rights and Economic Power* (University of Illinois Press, 2009).

patient care as "awful," and stating that, "I know if I were really very sick, I would not have wanted to be there."[43]

By late 1966, Taborian Hospital was on the verge of bankruptcy and having difficulties even meeting payroll. Sales of Taborian's insurance had plummeted due to profound unemployment in the region. Tufts responded in two ways. First, from its own grant and university funds, it provided a loan to Taborian Hospital to avert the immediate financial crisis. Second, Geiger suggested to OEO that it should fund hospital care for blacks in the area through a grant requiring the two ailing community hospitals to be merged into a new Mound Bayou Community Hospital with adequate resources. OEO agreed to provide federal funding for free hospitalization in Mound Bayou to poor people in Bolivar and surrounding counties, and the health center would provide primary care, both curative and preventative, for the poor of north Bolivar County.[44]

In addition to securing additional funding for health care in Bolivar County, Geiger saw additional advantages to this agreement: "By tying the Tufts Health Center project to some desperately-needed Federal assistance for two Mississippi institutions ... I made it very nearly impossible for the Mississippi governor and others in the power structure to oppose the Tufts project." OEO asked Geiger to write a grant proposal to effect a hospital merger and fund a new community hospital in Mound Bayou. The proposal mandated that, in accordance with its goal of "maximum feasible participation of the poor," in order to receive the federal grant the two hospitals must merge and be governed by a newly constituted community board representative of members of its target population—the rural poor—instead of the leaders of the fraternal orders. As Geiger remembered, the fraternal leaders "totally could not see why there had to be a community board, why the Knights and Daughters of Tabor didn't continue to run it," and protested the creation of the new board, even though the hospitals faced bankruptcy without the proposed federal aid. Meharry's Matthew Walker, who had a long standing relationship with the Taborian leadership, acted as an intermediary. He reported to Dr. John Frankel of the OEO that "Taborian rejected your proposal," because "they did not want to turn the hospital into a community hospital. They pointed out that the organization's members were insistent that 'We don't want to give our hospital away'." In an effort to mollify the situation, OEO permitted the two fraternal societies to appoint one-third of the board of directors of the new Mound Bayou Community Hospital,

---

[43] Geiger Letter to Dr. Alexander Robinson, June 25, 1966, *JGC*; Beito, "Black Fraternal Hospitals in Mississippi Delta, 1942–1967," 129–30; Hatch notes, *JHC*.
[44] Jack Geiger notes, *JGC*.

with the remaining positions to be drawn from members of the target community. A deal was reached.[45]

Although certainly necessary if there was going to be readily available hospital care for health center patients if they should need it, in many ways, this arrangement pleased no one and sowed the seeds of future conflict between the health center and the new community hospital. Geiger and Hatch objected to the new board, which they saw as being dominated by those with ties to the fraternal orders and town elite, and as not being inclusive enough of either the members or the interests of the larger Bolivar County community. The fraternal leaders were upset that they now had to share control of what they still perceived as "their" hospital, and, without the ability to charge their previous fees for hospital service, they also saw their memberships decline rapidly. Finally, leaders of Mound Bayou's governing elite (aided, somewhat ironically, by the governor and other white state leaders), who dominated the new hospital board, began to argue that now that OEO was funding the Mound Bayou Community Hospital (MBCH), the proposed Tufts–Delta Health Center was unnecessary. Federal funding, they asserted, should go only to the community hospital—and be controlled by them, not outsiders from Massachusetts. As Geiger later lamented, "The effort to rescue and stabilize the hospitals had thus inadvertently created an instrument that could be used to compete for control of the Tufts–Delta Health Center."[46]

Despite these tensions, the plans went forward for both the new hospital and the health center to open. The conflicts that had characterized the planning of the center were not over, and friction between the health center and its numerous critics would continue for years to come; but Geiger, Hatch, and the team that they assembled were finally able to begin delivering services to the impoverished clientele in the Delta. Because of the urgent need, Geiger and his staff of what became the Tufts–Delta Health Center began offering clinical programs in 1966 in temporary quarters in a rented five-room church parsonage while its permanent facility was being constructed.

---

[45] Geiger Letter to Dr. Alexander Robinson, June 25, 1966, *JGC*; DeJong, "Plantation Politics," 261; Beito, "Black Fraternal Hospitals in the Mississippi Delta," 138–39; Interview with H. Jack Geiger by Robert Korstad and Neil Boothby; Letter from Dr. Matthew Walker to Dr. John Frankel, OEO, June 1, 1967, Series 1, Subseries 1, Box 8, Folder 57, *DHC*.

[46] DeJong, "Plantation Politics," 261; Beito, "Black Fraternal Hospitals in the Mississippi Delta," 138–39; Interview with H. Jack Geiger by Robert Korstad and Neil Boothby; Letter from John Hatch to John Frankel, OEO, December 15, 1966, *JHC*; Jack Geiger notes, *JGC*.

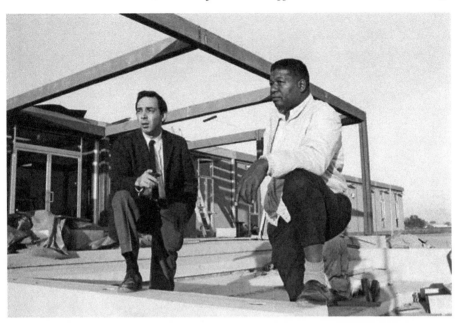

FIGURE 1.1 Jack Geiger and John Hatch overlooking the construction of the Tufts-Delta Health Center (Photo courtesy of Dan Bernstein, private collection).

It was strange to the poor to be treated with dignity, but it felt good.
PEARLIA B. ROBINSON[1]

The status of the poor cannot be changed significantly until a redistribution of power occurs.
JOHN HATCH[2]

2

Community Organizing

BEFORE ANY HEALTH services could be delivered by Tufts in Mississippi, ground work had to be laid with the local community. Therefore, in order to first prepare for, and eventually coordinate, the various programs of the Tufts–Delta Health Center across the rural, 500 square-mile area of north Bolivar County, John Hatch embarked on a massive community organizing effort during his first year in the county. To do so, he consulted with a number of prominent black Mississippians, including Owen Brooks and Amzie Moore, to get both their support for the proposed health center and elicit their advice on how best to proceed. Moore, from Cleveland, Bolivar County's urban center, was a World War II veteran who returned to the Mississippi Delta determined both to resist Jim Crow and to insulate himself from its ravages. He became one of the Delta's most successful black businessmen, owning a store, a gas station, and numerous properties. During the 1950s and 1960s, he was active in the state NAACP, and worked as a liaison between SNCC (Student Nonviolent Coordinating Committee) volunteers and the local population during Freedom Summer. Brooks,

[1] Pearl B. Robinson, "The Community Part in Health Center Program," presented at the 97th Annual Meeting of the American Public Health Association and Meeting of Related Organizations, Nov. 10–14, 1969, Philadelphia, Penn. Excerpted in "Voices from the Past," *American Journal of Public Health* (September 11, 2014): e3.
[2] John W. Hatch, "Discussion of Group Practice in Comprehensive Healthcare Centers," *Bulletin of the New York Academy of Medicine*, second series, Vol. 44, No. 11, (November 1968): 1375–77.

a Boston native, was the head of the Delta Ministry, the largest civil rights organization in the state, which focused primarily on improving the economic plight of black
Mississippians.[3]

Along with the counsel of Moore and Brooks, Hatch sought to identify local
leaders, the traditional spokespeople of the Delta's black community, to get them to
support the proposed health center and its programs, and serve as ambassadors for
the center's staff to make inroads with members of the small, scattered, communities of the county, such as Rosedale, Duncan, Round Lake, and Alligator. These tiny
hamlets, and the rural plantations that surrounded them, were home to over 10,000
black residents in the mid-1960s. Although the health center would be located in the
all-black town of Mound Bayou, the main targets of the health center's programs
were those who lived in these much more remote areas, who had almost no access
to healthcare programs. Vital to the success of these outreach efforts was the involvement of the traditional "gatekeepers of the black community," as Hatch called
them—deacons and ministers, principals and school teachers, landowners and businessmen. Initially, many of these gatekeepers were not very enthusiastic about the
health center, in part due to a learned skepticism of outsiders promising aid to the
black community while delivering either nothing, or worse, exploitation. Ministers
feared that opening their doors to representatives of the health center, which they
knew was not a popular institution among the white community, might bring about
some retribution from powerful whites. Many members of the black elite also were
tied closely to the Knights and Daughters of Tabor, and feared that the proposed
health center was a threat to both the Taborian Hospital and the financial stability of the fraternal organization itself. Still others, including many school teachers
and principals, saw the health center as an outgrowth of the civil rights movement
(which it certainly was), led by outsiders, and were wary that any involvement with
the Tufts–Delta Health Center could jeopardize their employment, which was still
subject to the whims of all-white school boards.[4]

Despite a great deal of reluctance, a number of churches did open their doors
to representatives of the health center, and—predictably—ministers were some of
the most important contacts that the health center made in opening doors to the
community. Of all the ministers who aided Hatch in his community outreach,
none was more valuable than Reverend H. Y. Ward of Mound Bayou, who had
pastored churches throughout the area. "I first met Rev. Ward during early spring
1966," recalled Hatch. "My objective during this period was to learn about the
social patterns of black people in Bolivar County. . . . I wanted better information

[3] Cobb, *The Most Southern Place on Earth*, 211, 241; Dittmer, *Local People*, 365.
[4] DeJong, "Plantation Politics," 265; Hatch Narrative, *JHC*.

about people living on plantations." Reverend Ward was a long-time member of both the Bolivar County Baptist Convention and the Knights and Daughters of Tabor, two of the most important local institutions for Bolivar County's black population. He was able to help Hatch identify and meet people who held positions of influence and authority—often in informal ways—within the Delta's black neighborhoods. Hatch soon learned that traveling throughout the county with Reverend Ward not only opened doors to black families who might not have been willing to meet with him, but also gave him access to plantations controlled by whites who would never have permitted Hatch to enter on his own. "I was riding with Rev. Ward to visit people he knew on the Bobo plantation," remembered Hatch. "The gate to the company store was open. A very large warning sign informing trespassers that voter registration workers were not allowed in on the Bobo property caused concern. I asked Rev. Ward, 'Might it be safer to go elsewhere?' He said, 'Oh, that does not mean us.' He explained that we were on God's business and God wants us to do what we can to feed his sheep. Rev. waved at the large white man carrying a pistol on his hip and kept driving. I was pleased to know about being on God's business, and even more pleased to be riding with a local pastor with easy access to the area."[5]

Reverend Ward proved to be an invaluable asset to Hatch, organizing meetings and promoting the virtues of the health center's pilot programs, such as home nursing and health education programs, and what was planned for the future. Reverend Ward later recalled "going around to the county, letting people know what's happening, what's coming to Mound Bayou as a place for health. From there I'd work just six, eight, nine months by myself, going across this county, have meetings with different churches and ministers across this county; the schools—Duncan school, Alligator school. . . . Meetings all over, all over."[6] Often because of Reverend Ward's insistence, other ministers also opened their churches to Hatch and members of the Tufts–Delta Health Center. Churches were vital centers for rural African Americans of the Delta—even among those who might not be especially religious—because they were centers of both community and communication for people isolated from many aspects of the modern world. The church provided both spiritual uplift and temporal support; deacons and deaconesses held high status in the community and often mediated local disputes. The physical church building was also essential to local black communities as a meeting place for all types of activities, because it was often the only large structure in a given area to be owned and controlled by African Americans and was located in a spot with which everyone was familiar.

---

[5] Hatch Narrative, *JHC*.
[6] John Hatch interview with Rev. H.Y. Ward, Southern Historical Collection.

Indeed, many Delta blacks tended to use the name of their closest church to identify where they lived, even if they were not a parishioner.

Hatch and his outreach staff traveled to churches throughout the county to explain the center's programs and recruit people for the health associations he envisioned. These associations, he hoped, would be established throughout north Bolivar County to provide the center with both insight into the needs of the people and to help administer its programs. These associations would help fill the Office of Economic Opportunity (OEO) mandate for "maximum feasible participation" of the poor that the health center's grant required, but, more importantly to Geiger and Hatch, the health associations would be vital mechanisms in empowering local people to set health priorities for themselves and their communities. Once established, the local health associations would elect representatives to a health council for all the communities in north Bolivar County, which would be the liaison between the Tufts–Delta Health Center and the people it served. Geiger and Hatch envisioned the health council as eventually serving as the governing board of the health center.

Central to Hatch's vision for the health associations was identifying and working through nontraditional leaders in the community, people who—because they were poor, illiterate, or female—had previously been excluded from positions of authority and decision-making. Hatch sought out people who had earned the respect of their neighbors through their actions, and whose voices held weight within their communities. "We were also systematically looking at relationships," recalled Hatch. "In time, you began to identify some people who related to some people in the population more strongly than others. Some would relate to older folks, younger folks, so forth. We'd just sort of make note of who was at the meeting and we kind of know that if we wanted to tap this population, here's the person." Nor were they looking for people with any specific healthcare expertise. According to Geiger, they were looking for "problem solvers and helpers, rather than health people."[7]

It took Hatch almost a year of knocking on doors, speaking at churches and schools, and organizing meetings throughout the county before the first health associations were finally established in 1967. One of the main difficulties that Hatch and his outreach team faced as they traveled throughout the county trying to develop the health associations was that they were initially talking about a service that did not yet exist, because the health center had yet to open its doors for doctor–patient medical care. The bigger problem, however, continued to be the difficulty of involving those community members who had traditionally been excluded from

---

[7] Interview with John Hatch and Jack Geiger by Tom Ward, June 27, 2012 (private; in possession of the author); Sobelson, "Participation, Power, and Place," 61.

leadership positions in active roles in the development of the health associations. "We initiated meetings in schools, churches, and large halls to talk about hopes, dreams and ways to help improve health," recalled Hatch. "These orientation meetings were well attended. We spoke of the need for preventative health and health maintenance as well as for sick care. In Q&A after each presentation, it was clear that people deferred to preachers, teachers, church elders and other higher status people."[8]

Undeterred, Hatch, with the assistance of gatekeepers like Reverend Ward, continued to seek out local leaders in small black communities of the Delta. Reverend Ward introduced Hatch to Joe Clemons, a tractor driver on a plantation in the small town of Alligator. Clemons was exactly the type of person Hatch sought to ally himself with in the local communities—not a preacher, teacher, or businessman who had traditionally spoken for the black community because of his status, but someone who had earned the respect of his neighbors through years of work and friendship. After the men were introduced, Clemons agreed to help Hatch make contact with other influential people in the Alligator community. A week later, Hatch met with about thirty people at a local church. Afterward Clemons came up to Hatch and told him, "We think you are mighty smart to be working for big people. You talk like a learned man. We here in Alligator want to be guided by you." Hatch was crushed, feeling again that he was unable to connect with people in the ways that he needed. "I had heard words like this before," he recalled. "I understood the dynamics, but these words were the type of response black people reserved for white folk when they tried to communicate with black people. . . . What I learned was that being black was not much help in overcoming reluctance to risk stating true thoughts. I left wondering if I could establish meaningful dialogue, how long it might take, and what pathways I might best follow."[9]

This difficulty in breaking through to many locals and convincing them that he wanted their input, their ideas, and their involvement in the health center's programs was a tremendous obstacle for Hatch to overcome in getting the community support he and Geiger knew would be central to the success of the health center. Searching for ways to better involve those who did not speak up in larger gatherings, Hatch consulted with Jim Taylor, the associate director of community health action at the health center. Taylor suggested that instead of the mass meetings, Hatch should meet people in a more comfortable social environment. Hatch therefore began to ask some people he had identified as community leaders if they would host smaller gatherings in their homes—or under a shade tree on the plantation—about issues

---

[8] Hatch narrative, *JHC*.
[9] Hatch narrative, *JHC*.

they considered important to their neighborhood. This strategy proved helpful in gaining insight into the social structure of communities, because the hosts usually invited persons with whom they were already comfortable talking. In these small gatherings, those who often had not been comfortable speaking in more formal settings did participate, and Hatch was finally able to make breakthroughs in getting the input of many "nontraditional" leaders of the community.[10]

Another way Hatch tried both to include those whose voices were rarely heard and keep traditional leaders from dominating the health associations was by structuring the organizational meetings around specific issues. Without traditional leaders dominating the committees, Hatch believed, new voices could be heard, and new leaders would emerge. He worked especially hard to include women, who historically had been excluded from most decision-making positions in the Delta. For example, a committee was established on the needs of young mothers, which, of course, attracted young women, and also did not appeal to older men who were usually in charge of committees. "The deacons didn't show up [to the] young mothers' committee," remembered Hatch with a smile, which was exactly the idea. He understood that women would be important consumers of the health center's services, and their input and involvement would, be central to its success. Hatch also saw women as vital connectors in the community who could bring others to the center. One local woman whose help Hatch sought was Ethel Sheraton Dennis, who owned and operated a beauty salon that was patronized by most of the black professional and business women in Bolivar County, most of whom were also very influential in the county's churches and fraternal societies. "Her help in meeting powerful but less visible women was extremely valuable in gaining insight into women's role in the social order," recalled Hatch. "Through her, I was able to visit women in their homes. . . . Her endorsement shortened the time required to build rapport."[11]

Although Mrs. Dennis came from the traditional black elite leadership class, one woman who emerged as an important leader in the health associations did not. Pearlia B. Robinson, or "Miss Pearlie," as most people called her, was from the tiny hamlet of Round Lake, about a mile from the Mississippi River. "She was maybe 5 feet tall and maybe weighed 250. Close to God," remembered Hatch. "A very bright person, but, you know, not lettered, as was the case of many people in the Delta at that time. . . . Pearl was a sleeper . . . a likable community activist who could speak to anybody, and do it very well." Hatch first came into contact with Miss Pearlie at the health association orientation meeting in the town of Gunnison.

---

[10] Hatch narrative, *JHC*.
[11] Ward interview with Hatch and Geiger.

She stood up and said, "You people say you want to hear what our needs are and start where we would like to start. But you talk about babies all the time. What's happening in this community is old people who expected to be nurtured by their families, those families are in Chicago and St. Louis and Detroit. And our old people are being neglected." Her message was not what Hatch and the other members of the health center team had expected, but it was exactly what they wanted and needed to hear—the real concerns of the members of the community, not the concerns that the leaders of the Tufts–Delta Health Center had brought with them from Boston. "Miss Pearl got it," recalled Hatch. "She understood the rhetoric—'We want to start where you are' and all that stuff." Hatch responded to her appeal at Gunnison, and at other health association meetings, that something be done for the elderly in north Bolivar County. "While the center's initial goal was to deal with children and infant mortality," he later wrote, "concerns from the community like those of Miss Pearlie B. forced the center to adapt, and expand the types of services that it needed to develop and provide." The position of "Coordinator of Services to the Elderly" was therefore created at the Tufts–Delta Health Center, and Miss Pearlie was hired to fill the position. She proved to be one of the center's most important activists, not only in regards to elder care, but on a whole host of community issues and concerns.[12]

As Miss Pearlie had put forth in Gunnison, one of the main issues to emerge in the organizational meetings for the health center, whether among large groups in churches or small groups under shade trees, was that "health care was not the issue of greatest concern to most people as they understood help," recalled Hatch. "While most had been poor all of their lives, they were now worse off because of the displacement of farm labor by weed control agents and cotton harvesting equipment."[13] Instead, Hatch heard about the need for clean water to drink, fuel to heat their shacks, livable housing, pest control, child care, and jobs. People told stories of sewage running through front yards, and children drinking water out of drainage ditches. Other communities complained of their inability to clothe children properly for school. Repeatedly, Hatch heard that the most pressing issue for the black people of Bolivar County was hunger. "Health services are fine, and what you talk about sounds good," said one participant at an organizational meeting, "but for the love of God, can you share some food?"[14]

---

[12] Ward interview with Hatch and Geiger; Hatch narrative, *JHC*.

[13] Hatch narrative, *JHC*.

[14] H. Jack Geiger, "Community Control—or Community Conflict? *Bulletin of the National Tuberculosis and Respiratory Disease Association* (November, 1969): 4–10.

"There were two or three other priorities that came ahead of health as we ordinarily define it," Geiger recalled. "These were food, jobs, housing, and then maybe education. Health was fourth or fifth on the list.... What people were telling us was, 'We have a somewhat different set of priorities; what are you going to do about it?'" Geiger and Hatch both viewed health care as an entry point to dealing with other issues of poverty and inequality in the Mississippi Delta, but they soon began to understand that the issues that the local population saw as most important also could work as entrees to their health care programs. Therefore, as the health associations began to take shape around the county, each one developed its own priorities, and the health center's staff worked to help them achieve their specific goals. By allowing the local associations not only to have a voice, but also to set the priorities for their communities, the health center both empowered these new health associations and made their leaders more willing to work with the health center on issues that it found important. Geiger contrasted this effort with what he saw as a lack of community buy-in at Columbia Point, where Tufts came in with its plan and relied much less on local leadership and decision-making. Instead of a "top-down" approach, in which the health center told the local communities what they needed and what it would do for them, in Bolivar County Geiger and Hatch were flexible enough to allow locals to identify the most pressing needs for their communities, and then work with them through the auspices of the Tufts–Delta Health Center to try and achieve the goals they all sought. As one local man stated at an organizational meeting, "I didn't have the slightest idea of what can be done through a *health* project. Listening to Brother Hatch here talk about how we can improve ourselves gives me a little more courage to take back home with me."[15]

The long process of identifying local leaders and building the health associations from the "bottom up" caused Hatch some tension with his federal funders. "During the first year there was pressure from the OEO to organize a group able to represent the citizens of north Bolivar County," he recalled. "Our decision to build from the bottom up took more time than the usual top-down type organizational model ..., [but] the top-down model would've affirmed the perception of community held by those already identified as persons able to speak for the poor and less articulate. The problem with the model was that these leaders often had little interaction with the poor, and seldom solicited their opinion; although they speak in the interest of the poor, it is their perception of the needs of poor people that is more often expressed." Hatch feared that creating the health associations quickly, as OEO wanted, would have resulted in the traditional spokespersons—middle class blacks and some

---

[15] Geiger, "Community Control—or Community Conflict? 8–9; Hall, "A Stir of Hope in Mound Bayou," 78.

whites—speaking for north Bolivar County's poor, instead of the poor speaking for themselves.[16]

Therefore, Hatch and his staff continued knocking on doors, identifying people he thought would be effective leaders, and organizing on what he called the "micro-level." He stated, "You'd inevitably find people, some of whom tended to invite people just like them" to discuss developing a health association. In Shelby, Clementine Murray was approached by health center staff to start a health association in her community. She agreed to serve as the Shelby health association's first chairman, and set off to recruit members. "I had, in the beginning, about five or six people who thought this was a good idea and they followed me. We didn't have a meeting place, so we started meeting at the church. And, finally, one or two more would drift in, until we had about 15, I guess," she later remembered. "We just put out flyers in the community saying this was an important meeting and asking the peoples to come out. Because then we were trying to get people started out to try to get the association organized; nominating peoples, and getting peoples interested in what to do, and see how well they did in getting them elected as officers of the health association." Throughout north Bolivar County, local leaders like Clementine Murray helped establish ten local health associations by 1967—on the "bottom-up" model. Each health association emerged out of the interest groups that Hatch had helped develop in the individual communities on issues such as maternal and child health, elderly care, environmental needs, youth development, and employment opportunities. The chairs of these small committees served as the core leadership of each health association, and all the members of the association elected an association president and other officers.[17]

Having established health associations throughout the health center's target area—in the towns of Alligator, Beulah, Duncan, Gunnison, Marigold, Mound Bayou, Round Lake, Rosedale, Symonds, & Shelby—Hatch then sought to create a health council to act as an umbrella organization to coordinate the activities of all ten health associations and serve as an advisory body to the Tufts–Delta Health Center. To develop the health council, Hatch asked each local health association to select three people to sit on the council planning committee; to ensure that different views from each community were represented, he required that each delegation include at least one member of the opposite sex and at least one member under age 30. The health council was modeled on the governance structure of the Baptist Church, an institution most every African American in the Mississippi Delta understood

---

[16] John Hatch Narrative, *JHC*.

[17] John Hatch Narrative, *JHC*; Interview with John Hatch by Robert Korstad and Neal Boothby; Mrs. Clementine Murray Interview, Delta Health Center Tapes (Disk 1, Reels 5–6 and 5–7).

and respected, whether they were church-going folks or not. As the Baptist Church
Association provides a governance structure while still allowing for the autonomy
of its affiliated churches, the North Bolivar County Health and Civic Improvement
Council, as it was officially incorporated, created a structure for its auxiliary health
associations while still allowing each a great deal of freedom to manage issues in
their local area. The council also adapted electoral methods from the black church,
in which members did not have to vote publicly against family members or friends.
Each of the ten health associations was represented by one member on the health
council, elected by the members of his or her local association.[18]

The North Bolivar County Health Council (NBCHC), as the North Bolivar
County Health and Civic Improvement Council, Inc., was commonly known, was
formally organized in August of 1968. Council meetings were held twice monthly,
on the second and fourth Sunday afternoons, at the Tufts–Delta Health Center
in Mound Bayou; meetings were open to anyone who wanted to attend, but only
the representatives could vote on measures. The meetings always included some sort
of presentation by health center staff or an invited guest. Presentations were made
by doctors, nurses, and other professional staff concerning issues such as social services, pharmaceuticals, and environmental health. Some issues did not deal directly
with health care, but went directly to the council's mission of civic improvement.
For example, the center's psychologist, Dr. Florence Halpern, conducted sessions on
early child learning in school, while the center's lawyer talked about ways in which
people could protect themselves when making major purchases, and a housing spe-
cialist discussed how poor people with limited income could build and improve
their housing. In addition to the presentations, reports from the individual health
associations were given at the council meetings. Here, representatives shared both
the successes and struggles of their community association, and looked to both the
center's staff and their fellow council members for advice.[19]

Once the not-for-profit charter was signed by the governor in 1969, the North
Bolivar County Health Council became eligible for OEO funding and was able to
hire its own executive director—Dave Caldwell of Symonds—a secretary, and ten
part-time staff. The health council's offices were housed in a three-room suite in
the Tufts–Delta Health Center. Initially, the council focused on programs it saw as
vital to both health and civic improvement, such as transportation, low-cost housing, and legal services for the poor. Transportation was a major issue for both the

---

[18] John Hatch, "Self-Help and Consumer Participation in the Development of the Health Care System," unpublished manuscript, Box 42, Folder 314, *DHC*; John Hatch Narrative, *JHC*; Sobelson, "Participation,
Power, and Place," 58.

[19] North Bolivar County Health Report, n.d. Box 42, Folder 310, *DHC*.

Tufts–Delta Health Center and the North Bolivar County Health Council because many people in rural Bolivar County had no way to get to Mound Bayou to receive care at the health center. Initially, the health center tried to meet the transportation needs with rental cars, but the costs were unsustainable. The health council pointed out that every (black) public school in north Bolivar County hired black contractors to provide school bus service. These buses were busy between 7:00 and 8:30 a.m. and between 3:00 and 4:30 p.m., but then sat idle the rest of the time. The health council negotiated with these contractors to provide an efficient, low-cost bus service to link the health center with pick-up points in the surrounding communities served by the health associations. The council hired Morris Bell, a former army sergeant who ran a motor pool, to oversee the program. This service provided both access to medical services at the health center, and economic mobility for both workers and shoppers.[20]

Along with the transportation system, which was a boon to the poor of north Bolivar County, the health council also began legal services for those in need. The council contracted with a senior corporate lawyer in Jackson to be available for consultations one day a week at the health center, and a recent law school graduate to handle more routine matters. The legal aid usually focused on individual issues, such as access to food stamps or other federal welfare programs. "Our lawyer has only been part time but he is doing wonderful work," reported the council. "People have been helped out of trickey [*sic*] deals. And he helps people with papers on housing and land." The lawyers also worked with the local communities on issues such as getting local governments to provide paved roads, streetlights, garbage removal, and water and sewer systems in their areas.[21]

Housing was another focus of the council's leadership—both providing improvements to current housing, usually in conjunction with the health center's environmental health division, or working for the development of low-cost housing in the county. One issue that emerged as the health council began to work to improve housing was the systematic discrimination from banks in providing loans to Bolivar County's black citizens. Blacks in Bolivar County suffered from crushing poverty, and banks were understandably unwilling to provide mortgages for those they feared would be unable to pay. Indeed, the health center's Resource Development Unit found that in 1970, "Out of the 51 applications

---

[20] "The Delta Health Center Digest" (October 1969), 8–10, *DHC*; H. Jack Geiger, "Community-Oriented Primary Care: A Path to Community Development," *American Journal of Public Health* Vol. 92, No. 11 (November 2002): 1713–16.

[21] "The Delta Health Center Digest" (October 1969), 8–10; Letter from Andrew James to B. J. Stiles, Director, RFK Fellows, Jan. 5, 1970, *DHC*; North Bolivar County Health Report, n.d., Box 42, Folder 310, *DHC*; Geiger, "Community Control—or Community Conflict?" 8–9.

submitted through this office to the Farmers Home Administration for individual home loans, only 15 were approved. The above figure emphasizes the fact that there are still no rural housing programs to meet the needs of families earning less than $3000 a year. This looms large as a factor since the average income is much less than $1,500 per year."[22]

Poverty, however, was not the only obstacle. As was true across the nation, African Americans were regularly denied Federal Housing Administration (FHA)-backed mortgages, and, therefore, left to contract sales or other unscrupulous loans in order to try to finance homes. In Mound Bayou and throughout the Mississippi Delta, Geiger remembered, "blacks couldn't get a mortgage to build a house, except either with a white co-signer and all of the costs that came with that, or under the table at usurious interest rates of one kind or another, and the whole set of socioeconomic problems that went with that." In order to try to alleviate the difficulties of African Americans getting mortgages—or even loans for appliances or cars—John Hatch decided that the health center could leverage the money it was bringing into the region to get more equitable service for its black citizens. He and health council leaders went to a number of local banks and explained that the Tufts–Delta Health Center had a cash flow of two million dollars a year, which was currently being handled by a Memphis bank. They explained that they would rather have the money handled locally, but would only do business with a bank that agreed to open a branch in Mound Bayou, employ black people as tellers, and give mortgages to black people—especially those on the health center and health council staffs with secure jobs—on the same terms as anyone else. Geiger recalled that "the smallest, previously most racist bank in the region, the Bank of Bolivar County," agreed to the deal, "because whatever kind of trouble they had with black, they didn't have with green." As a result of this intervention, local staff members obtained mortgages to build modest new homes, and the health associations obtained mortgages to buy buildings for satellite centers.[23]

The economic impact of the health center on Bolivar County was significant, both in the influx of federal money into the county and the employment opportunities that the Tufts–Delta Health Center provided. The 1960s saw a loss of over 40,000 agricultural jobs in the Mississippi Delta, as mechanization and chemicals dramatically reduced the need for sharecrop labor; black unemployment in the region hovered around 75 percent. Few new employment opportunities replaced the

---

[22] "Progress Reports, 1971—Division of Community Health Action," *DHC*.

[23] Interview with H. Jack Geiger by Robert Korstad and Neil Boothby; Geiger, "Community-Oriented Primary Care: A Path to Community Development," 1714. For more on the difficulties that African Americans had securing home loans in twentieth-century America, see Ta-Nehisi Coates, "The Case for Reparations," *The Atlantic* (June 2014): 54–71.

thousands of lost agricultural jobs, and most of the former sharecroppers had very little education and few, if any, marketable skills off the plantation. As the *Boston Globe* reported on Bolivar County in 1967, "Many [black] parents have never attended school. Mississippi has no compulsory school attendance laws and . . . [many] children . . . have never attended school regularly. The Negroes know little beyond picking cotton, many can neither read nor write, and there are few jobs even if they are trained."[24] Jobs and education for the Delta's poor were, therefore, major concerns of both the health council and the health center.

One of the immediate impacts of the Tufts–Delta Health Center on Bolivar County was its ability, with its federal funding, to provide a number of jobs for members of its target population, with an emphasis on hiring the people who were often seen as "unemployable" because of their lack of skills and education. By 1970, programs affiliated with the Tufts–Delta Health Center and funded by OEO were the largest employers of blacks in Bolivar County, providing over 180 jobs. Although all the professional staff initially came from outside of the area, Geiger and Hatch worked hard to fill as many staff positions as possible with locals. Geiger recalled being overwhelmed by the demand: "We were living in trailers near the center site. One morning I got up to find 15 people on my doorstep. They heard about [a] job opening and waited all night to apply." With so many people in need, one of the most difficult tasks for Geiger was trying to determine who would get a coveted position at the health center, and who would be left unemployed. "At the entry level jobs in particular, we had probably fifteen or twenty applicants for every position," he recalled. "How do you choose? Here were jobs where almost everyone had the basic qualifications." Previously, much of the wage employment in and around Mound Bayou had been controlled by the local black elite and determined through connections. John Hatch recalled that "patronage was a way of life [when we arrived in Mound Bayou]. Under the direction of the Health Center employment became fairer and more equitably based." For example, an announcement for a job as a truck driver might attract forty applications, and perhaps thirty-five applicants would meet the health center's criteria in terms of fitness and safety qualifications. In a region where a truck driving job would place a person in the top 10 percent of wage earners, competition was keen for such a position. After qualifications were determined, geography and good citizenship, along with social responsibility, need, and reputation were major determinants of staff selection.[25]

---

[24] "Tufts Plan: Negroes' Only Ray of Hope."

[25] North Bolivar County farm cooperative self-help nutritional program. Grant proposal (written by Hatch), 1972, *JHP*; L. C. Dorsey, "Dirt Dauber Nest, Socks Nailed Over Doorways, Salts, Prayer, and OTC's," unpublished manuscript, *DHC*; Geiger interview by Korstad and Boothby; Lefkowitz, *Community Health Centers*, 37; Hatch narrative, *JHC*.

Because jobs at the Tufts–Delta Health Center were so greatly sought, one of the early conflicts that emerged between the center's staff and the health council concerned the hiring procedures at the health center. "We were criticized for not providing more services, for not giving local people a chance," remembered John Hatch. "When one person was employed, some of the 40 odd others who applied for the job often felt mistreated." Many members of the health council were upset because they believed that the majority of the positions at the health center were being filled by people from Mound Bayou, while the rural people, who made up a larger percentage of the population, were being left out. In response, Geiger agreed to work with the council to improve hiring practices. From this meeting, the council members and health center leaders agreed that the council's personnel committee would take part in all hiring. As a result of these negotiations, the health council provided input on many of the employment decisions at the health center, and eventually even new professional staff were interviewed by the council's jobs committee. The council developed an interesting method for screening its applicants in order to try and make sure that positions were equitably distributed throughout the county, and that those most in need of jobs got them. In essence, the hiring recommendations were turned over to the local health associations, who tried to ascertain who from their communities had the best combination of need and fit for a particular position. "What they did, in a remarkable process," recalled Geiger, "[was] they would run through on basis of what they knew: 'Mrs. Smith's husband died and she has three young kids'. But someone else would say, 'Yeah, but she gets a lot of help from her brother in Detroit; he sends a check every month.' Then they would weigh relative need on the basis of what they knew, and they made the decisions as to jobs. . . . There was community consensus on who got work, in a way we could have never have done ourselves because we did not have access to that kind of information."[26]

In order to help fill the vacant positions at the Tufts–Delta Health Center from a largely uneducated and untrained workforce, the center's staff provided instruction in numerous fields for members of the local population. "It was necessary for us to train the people we need from our resident population," recalled Andrew James, who directed the health center's Division of Environmental Services. "Their education prevents them from taking advantage of some of the existing programs that are available. Some of these [people] can't even begin to think about filing an application for anything, even though they're eligible for it . . . it's just a lost cause.

---

[26] North Bolivar County farm cooperative self-help nutritional program. Grant proposal (written by John Hatch), 1972, *JHP*; North Bolivar County Health Report, n.d., Box 42, Folder 310, *DHC*; John Hatch Narrative, *JHC*; Geiger interview by Korstad and Boothby.

So training is the lifeblood of this center. What we are trying to do is train young people, young blacks, to introduce them to new disciplines in life."[27]

Intensive, short-term programs were therefore set up at the First Baptist Church in Mound Bayou to train people as medical record librarians, lab technicians, secretaries, nurses' aides, and for a host of other positions so they could work at the health center. Others were sent to an OEO program in Little Rock, Arkansas, for secretarial, clerical, and vocational training. Sarah Atkinson was a project analyst with OEO. "I think Mound Bayou was one of the first, if not the first [community health center], that started sending people to school, hiring local people," she recalled. "They were all supposed to hire local people, but it seemed to me that Mound Bayou put more effort into it than others did, because others would say 'we can't find anybody with the right qualifications.' In the meantime, Mound Bayou Health Center was paying for people to go to school to get those qualifications." Mrs. Clementine Murray had only an eighth grade education and was working as a maid in the Shelby Hospital when she entered the training program at the Tufts–Delta Health Center. "I started working in the training school for four months, in nurse aide training, and there I was very successful, and I accomplished a good bit through the nurse aides course," she recalled. "I was happy to be one of the employees of Tufts and I thought that my share toward poverty peoples would be as working as hard as I could on the job. . . . Now that I'm working on the staff, is one of the employees of Tufts as a nurses' aide, working in the surgery department, I have learned to overcome obstacles that I had never been faced with before, being very successful, and now being able to do that by myself."[28]

The economic impact that the Tufts–Delta Health Center had on the local economy cannot be overstated. As unemployment skyrocketed in the region with the machination of plantations, jobs for women like Mrs. Murray—if they could find anything at all—were usually limited to work as maids or cooks, paying perhaps $15 a week. Because of the training provided by the health center, in 1969, twenty-one of the health center's twenty-six nurses and nurses' aides were local people, and seventy-five county residents worked at the Tufts–Delta Health Center; the next year, of the center's 200 employees, 180 were Bolivar County natives. With the influx of federal dollars and training provided by the health center, new opportunities were open to many, despite limited skills or education. Irene Williams was one of the first local people hired at the Tufts–Delta Health Center. She had little

[27] Andy James Interview, Delta Health Center Tapes (Disk 1, Reel 5–5).

[28] Geiger, "Community-Oriented Primary Care: A Path to Community Development," 1715; Geiger interview by Korstad and Boothby; Tom Ward interview with Sarah Atkinson, January 16, 2013 (private, in possession of the author); Mrs. Clementine Murray Interview, Delta Health Center Tapes (Disk 1, Reels 5–6 and 5–7).

education and no skills other than picking cotton. Hired as a trainee, she received $50 per week and eventually became a nurse's aide. The federal dollars also impacted pay scales throughout the area. Before the health center opened, Taborian Hospital paid its staff less than any other hospital in Mississippi (the state where hospital pay was already the lowest in the country). But because of its federal funding, the hospital soon became one of the better paying institutions in the state as its salaries had to be in line with federal standards. The improved pay even encouraged some native Mississippians who had left the state to return. Frank Christian quit his job as a nurse at Chicago's Cook County Hospital and returned to Mississippi. "Many of us would never have left if there had been any way to make a living here," he remarked. "We knew there was a need for us here."[29]

Although jobs at the health center were a boon to those who got them, and to the local economy, which benefited from the increased spending power of those now employed, Geiger and Hatch believed that in order to produce lasting change among Mississippi's Delta poor, they needed not only to provide entry-level positions to those in current need, but to try to build a pathway out of poverty for generations to come. "We finally decided that we're not going to stay here the rest of our lives, and is this responsible behavior to come in here, raise expectations, turn stuff around, and then, you know, go merrily down the path?" remembered John Hatch. "We decided, no, it wouldn't be [right], and what we've got to do then, is to identify that cadre of bright, young people in this environment who can become our replacements."[30] Therefore, along with some of the basic job training programs the center sponsored to help fill its own needs, it also instigated a number of educational programs and opportunities to help introduce people to careers, not just jobs, and to create leaders for Bolivar County's next generation.

Because of the local population's educational inadequacies, in order to better prepare people for careers, the health center began a high school equivalency program for people to earn their GEDs. Taught by the center's professional staff—and often by their spouses, many of whom had experience in education—these evening classes proved to be extremely popular and inspired Geiger to add a college preparatory program to the center's offerings. Health center staff members Florence Halpern, Andrew James, Irene Easling, and John Hatch negotiated with the leaders of Mary Holmes Junior College, an African-American institution in West Point, Mississippi, about 150 miles east of Mound Bayou, to establish a satellite program on the health center's campus. Students could take classes taught at the health center

---

[29] Kim Lacy Rodgers, *Life and Death in the Delta* (New York: Palgrave MacMillan, 2006), 138; DeJong, "Plantation Politics," 263–64; "28-Year Partnership for Health in Mississippi," *Ebony* (April 1970): 48, 50, 52.
[30] Hatch interview by Korstad and Boothby.

and receive college credit at Mary Holmes. A dozen senior staff members moon-lighted without pay as instructors in the extension program, teaching courses in basic English, science, math, Black History, secretarial science, and early childhood development two nights a week at the health center. This "prep academy" program, as it often was called, provided opportunities that previously would have been un-thinkable for most of Bolivar County's black residents, and provided some of them with a pathway out of poverty. Roberta Martin joined the health center's staff in 1970 and took advantage of the educational opportunities it offered to become a licensed practical nurse (LPN). After she received her degree, she got a job at a local hospital, and, by 1974, she was making $100 a week as an LPN.[31]

In addition to classroom study, at the urging of the health council, the Tufts–Delta Health Center also began a work-study program for high school students to introduce them to possible careers in health care. After school and on Saturdays, students in the program trained at the health center and out in the field under pro-fessional supervision, helping in the lab, working in the pharmacy, digging sanitary latrines, driving wells, assisting physicians, or serving as nurses' aides. Along with the practical experience these students gained, the program put them in direct con-tact with black professionals who served as mentors. According to John Hatch, the value of these interactions for students was incalculable, given that they "provided a view of the world most considered beyond their reach. For most, the dream of professional careers was as distant a dream as a high school diploma, as Delta High School did not prepare graduates for the rigor required in most colleges. There were, however, very bright, highly motivated people able and willing to work long and hard as required to overcome deficits and reach for success." As a result of these interactions, he recalled that "parents unable to pursue advanced education them-selves, encouraged and supported their children toward health careers," and "the children of tenant farmers became nurses, sanitarians, lab technicians, and other health professionals."[32]

Geiger, Hatch, James, and other members of the center's staff also used their influence and connections to help get promising students from Bolivar County into college, and then graduate programs, across the nation. Hatch recalled that "The Mary Holmes/Tufts faculty persons lobbied friends, professors, and admin-istrators of institutions all over the nation toward opening opportunities to young people in the Delta. Within a year, youth from the Delta were studying at Atlanta

---

[31] North Bolivar County farm cooperative self-help nutritional program. Grant proposal (written by Hatch), 1972, *JHC;* "The Delta Health Center Digest" [Tufts–Delta Health Center newsletter], March/April 1970, Box 20, Folder 148, *DHC;* Geiger interview by Korstad and Boothby; Rodgers, *Life and Death in the Delta,* 138.

[32] Hall, "A Stir of Hope in Mound Bayou," 70; John Hatch Narrative, *JHC.*

University School of Social Work, Brandeis University, Tufts University School of
Medicine, [and] the University of Wisconsin." Aura Kruger, wife of center physician Leon Kruger, taught at the local high school during her time in Mound Bayou.
She became increasingly frustrated by the hopelessness brought on by the lack of
opportunities for her students, especially her most talented ones. Kruger, therefore,
reached out to a friend who was a dean at Brandeis University in her hometown of
Boston, to see whether the university would provide scholarships for some deserving
students from Bolivar County. Brandeis came through with three scholarships, and
the health center staff and local churches helped raise money for plane tickets and
warm clothes for the students. Because of the influence of the Krugers and others,
opportunities for talented students helped fulfill John Hatch's dream of providing
a new leadership class for Delta blacks, and, by 1975, the health center's educational
program had produced seven physicians, five doctorates in clinical sciences, two environmental engineers, six social workers, numerous nurses, and the first ten registered black sanitarians in Mississippi history.[33]

Willie B. Lucas was one of the first persons to take advantage of the educational
opportunities that the health center provided. Lucas was much better off than
most of Bolivar County's black population—he was college-educated and part of
the county's black elite (his brother, Earl, served as the long-time mayor of Mound
Bayou)—but his dream of becoming a physician seemed out of reach. He was
teaching high school chemistry in Mound Bayou when the health center opened.
Jack Geiger befriended Lucas and encouraged him to pursue medicine. Lucas recalled that Geiger then "set up an interview with me at Tufts. He flew me up to
Boston, and two or three weeks later I was in." After receiving his medical degree,
Dr. Lucas returned to Mound Bayou where he served at the health center in numerous positions—as a physician, medical director, and eventually executive director—
between 1977 and 1986, when he entered private practice in Greenville. "I enjoy my
work; I work hard; it's been a great life," reflected Lucas. "And I likely wouldn't have
gone to medical school . . . if that opportunity [of meeting Geiger and attending
Tufts] had not come along."[34]

Geiger encouraged Tufts to recruit more students like Lucas, and during the
1960s, 1970s, and 1980s a handful of black Mississippians, most of whom were
graduates of tiny Tougaloo College in Jackson, enrolled at Tufts Medical School,
in what became known as the school's "Mound Bayou initiative." Geiger asked the

[33] Jo Ivester, *The Outskirts of Hope: A Memoir of the 1960s Deep South* (Berkeley, Calif.: She Writes Press, 2015),
134–38; John Hatch Narrative, *JHC*; Dittmer, *The Good Doctors*, 234.

[34] Dittmer, *The Good Doctors*, 234–35; Dorsey, "Dirt Dauber Nest, Socks Nailed Over Doorways, Salts, Prayer,
and OTC's"; Bruce Morgan, "Up from Mississippi," *Tufts Medicine* Vol. 62, No. 2 (Spring 2003): 16–25.

dean at Tufts to set up "a separate admissions program to the medical school for the communities or regions we serve, and it is going to have a separate admissions committee, and you will set aside seven or eight—I forget what number of places—and they agreed." Geiger and his staff were active in identifying potential students. "We found them from here and from neighboring counties and some from Jackson," he recalled. "In that first year five black students, three of them from this county, were admitted to Tufts Medical School. With that, we set up as part of the health center a formal office of education."[35]

At the time the relationship began, Tufts had very few minority students, and many of its recruits from Mississippi had never even left the state before traveling the 1,500 miles to Boston. Malcolm Taylor, who graduated from Tufts Medical School in 1973, was one of only five black students in his class, but found that the network of black Mississippians at the school already had created a support team in New England. Charles Cook, who was told by the University of Mississippi that he was "not medical school material," followed Taylor to Tufts, graduating in 1975. The support of other black Mississippians resulted in a successful atmosphere at Tufts, as all of the Mound Bayou initiative students graduated. As Geiger had hoped, many of these graduates, including Drs. Taylor and Cook, came home to practice. Taylor, a cardiologist, returned to Jackson, while Cook, after earning his master's degree in public health from Harvard, became assistant chief for disease control in the state. "It was home," he stated, and it was also where he was needed, given that it was "a state that perennially ranked near the bottom of the list when it came to public health and quality of medical care rankings."[36]

* * *

By 1970, the county's ten local health associations had 2,835 members who both cooperated with the Tufts–Delta Health Center's programs and instituted some of their own. The health associations were semiautonomous agencies that operated under the structure and guidelines of the North Bolivar County Health Council. Each local association held elections for its officers every two years, and each association had three delegates on the health council board of directors. Although the local associations had the freedom to focus on the specific needs of their communities, all were required to have the following standing committees: mother and child, home and community improvement, elderly, sickness, youth programs, and complaint.[37] Each local association met regularly—usually once or twice a month—to discuss the issues of the local community. The programs of the local health associations,

---

[35] Geiger interview by Korstad and Boothby; Morgan, "Up from Mississippi," 18–20.

[36] Geiger interview by Korstad and Boothby; Morgan, "Up from Mississippi," 17–18, 20–21, 25.

[37] John Hatch, "North Bolivar County farm cooperative self-help nutritional program grant proposal, 1972," *JHC*.

were often, but not always, carried out with assistance from the Tufts–Delta Health Center, and dealt with a wide variety of issues important to their communities. Angetta Soderberg was a representative from the Round Lake Health Association. "We have sick committees, and we have aged committees, we have home improvement committees," she recalled. "We try very hard to give the aged people and the children the very best that we can. We have given recreation to the older people . . ., we've had several teenage parties." She stated, however, that many of the services that the association delivered focused on the most basic needs of the community: "Like people getting bread out. People is hungry. And people don't have wood, and all that kind of stuff. We fund all that. . . . The people in the association usually buy their folks wood. They pay $.25 a month—this money stays in our own treasury—and it used to do such things that need to be done in the community."[38]

As in Round Lake, the other local health associations focused on a host of issues, most of which were not directly related to healthcare. Programs to provide food, fuel, and recreational activities were set up by all the health associations. The need for fuel—firewood—was one of the most pressing needs for many of the Delta poor. As a result of this need, the health associations—often working in conjunction with one another—bought firewood in bulk and then were able to deliver it to their members at discount rates.[39]

The lack of food, which, of course, also impacted health, was another pressing need that the health associations attempted to alleviate. The Duncan, Hushpuckena & New Africa Health Association began a hot lunch program that provided forty to fifty meals every Tuesday and Thursday to shut-in residents of their area, a program that was later adopted by other associations. "This program is very much needed in these communities because there are so many aged people living alone, no one to talk to, no one to prepare them a decent meal. They feel neglected and they are. We feel this is one way for them to have communication with one another, keep their minds together, forgetting some of their worries and be more healthy," remarked Pearlia B. Robinson, who ran the hot lunch program at Round Lake. Some of the associations made sure people were able to get needed government assistance in the form of food stamps and welfare, while others organized people to register to vote. The Gunnison, Perthshire & Waxhaw Association organized a number of recreational activities, including movies and trips for its members. Clothing drives, especially for school children, were held by a number of the associations, as were

---

[38] Richard Knox, "Hope Comes to Mound Bayou," *Boston Globe* (April 26, 1970); Angetta Soderberg Interview, Delta Health Center Tapes, Disk 1, Reel 5–8.

[39] North Bolivar County Health Report, n.d., Box 42, Folder 310, *DHC*.

educational programs for children and adults. Many of the associations held fish fries, barbeques, raffles, and picnics to raise money for emergency funds to be distributed to community members in the greatest need.[40]

As the health associations gained more members and developed more programs, access to physical locations where they could meet and provide services for their communities grew more difficult to obtain. Each association tried to rent or buy their own building as a contact center for their community—and also to serve as a satellite center of the Tufts–Delta Health Center. One obstacle was that OEO guidelines prohibited the use of federal funds to purchase buildings, so neither Tufts nor the health associations could use federal funds to purchase buildings for these centers. Clementine Murray was chair of the Shelby Health Association when it sought to acquire a contact center. She found a home for sale and sought donations for a down payment. She was able to raise $500, but the bank refused to give the association a mortgage. Undeterred, she worked directly with the seller who was willing to bypass the bank and work directly with Murray and the association. An agreement was reached to buy the house with $500 down and monthly installments of $65 for the next four and a half years. Murray then needed to raise funds to repair the building. Support from the community—both financial and in-kind—as well as volunteers from the health association and the Tufts–Delta Health Center who performed a good deal of the labor, eventually made the facility a reality. "I started out looking for pledges [to fix up the house], and I [got] about $600," she remembered. "I had two people of Shelby that gave me a check for $100; and check[s] [for] $50, $25 . . . and I had one store owner donate a brand new swing. . . . We found out that the floor was in such bad shape we couldn't put in no rug . . . so we had to go back and get underlayment to put on the floor before we could put down the rug. We found we couldn't put down tile because the tile was too high [priced]. . . . After we shown the first movie in there—we showed the children a movie—we found that the room was not big enough and we had to start tearing down again!"[41]

This arrangement was replicated at other contact centers throughout the county. John Hatch's agreement with the Bank of Bolivar County made it possible for some health associations to obtain regular mortgages to buy buildings for satellite centers. Because Tufts could not build its own facilities, the health associations usually rented the buildings to the health center for use during the day as satellite clinics—an arrangement that not only provided people with an avenue for health care without having to travel to Mound Bayou, but also helped the local health association pay off the building without violating OEO guidelines. At night, the buildings

[40] Progress Reports, 1971, Box 38, Folder 285, *DHC*.
[41] Mrs. Clementine Murray Interview.

functioned as community centers. These contact, or satellite, centers proved to be vital to the success of the local health associations and helped them attract new members. People could meet there to discuss problems in their town, and how to fix them. Barbara Brooks remembered that, "A lot of times you would run up upon raw sewage, and as workers we would encourage those people to stand up and attend their town meeting and voice their opinion and talk about certain grants that could be gotten to cover these raw sewers, these ditches, and cutting the grass, and they developed this program whereas they had this machine that would go and spray for mosquitoes, because in Mississippi mosquitoes are very bad."[42]

Along with being places to conduct association business and hold community meetings, the contact centers provided a space for community activities—especially for children and the elderly—in poor areas of the county that lacked any such programs. Centers regularly hosted movies and picnics, and all had a phone to use—often the only one in the area available to poor blacks. Contact centers were even used for weddings, reunions, and birthday parties.[43] John Hatch recalled the Round Lake Center, an old eight-room home bought for $3000, as one of his favorite places in the county:

> Sometimes on Saturdays the association invited blues men and women to sing and pick. Stories were told of fun times and good times in the shadows of oppression. At times, a clear beverage that seemed to liven things up was passed around. The fried fish was always the day's catch, and other foods were market fresh and superbly prepared. Young folks danced and old folks remembered when they could. Round Lake and other centers became centers of community-focused events that poor folks controlled.[44]

For the center's health professionals, these satellite facilities were also vital. Although much of the work being done by the local health associations did not seem to fit the traditional concept of health care, Geiger and his staff encouraged a broad interpretation of their health care mission in the Delta, and welcomed the disparate programs of the health associations. The staff of the Tufts–Delta Health Center, however, also worked to initiate and encourage more traditional health-care-related

---

[42] Geiger, "Community-Oriented Primary Care," 1774; Interview with Barbara Brooks and Jack Cartwright by Martha Minette in Rosedale, Mississippi (1999), Southern Historical Collection, UNC–Chapel Hill.

[43] Geiger, "Community-Oriented Primary Care," 1774; Report of Round Lake, Deeson, and Hill House Health Association, n.d. [1970], Box 42, Folder 311, *DHC*.

[44] John Hatch Narrative, *JHC*.

programs through the health associations, and the contact centers provided an important entrée into improving the health of Bolivar County' poor. These centers were places to conduct health education classes, well-child discussions, and group sessions with nurses and nutritionists from the health center—programs that many people would not have traveled to Mound Bayou to attend, but would go to if they were close to home. Doctors and nurses could provide basic evaluations at the satellite centers and identify those who needed to travel to Mound Bayou for further treatment at the health center or hospital. The satellite centers also served as transportation hubs for the health council's bus system, where people could get a ride to Mound Bayou. In addition to their benefits for health care delivery, these centers were also places where health center staff could discuss a host of other issues with the local population. Social workers came to the centers to help deal with family and child rearing concerns; environmental engineers conducted sessions on clean water and pest removal; financial advisors discussed strategies to secure loans for homes and large appliances; and lawyers provided legal aid.[45]

Child care soon emerged as another focus of the health associations. There was some child care at the Tufts–Delta Health Center, but it was what Dr. Aaron Shirley described as a "drop-in center," more than a complete day care facility. "When moms would come to the clinic and brought the children, even if the children weren't ill, we had a special place for kids for enrichment," he remembered. "For the first time a lot of the kids would see coloring books; people would read to them; and they'd have a chance to be part of a group. And that wasn't traditional." The drop-in facility at the health center was not sufficient to deal with the child care needs of the entire target population, however, and the health council sought to establish a more complete facility. With the help of an OEO grant, in September 1970 the health council opened its first a day care center at the contact center at Round Lake.[46]

To improve child care in the county, the health associations also looked to the federal Head Start program, which had been extremely controversial in Mississippi. A centerpiece of President Johnson's War on Poverty, Head Start was an OEO-funded program to provide preschool learning opportunities for poor children aged three to five years. Begun in 1966 as a summer project, it eventually was expanded to school-year programs in impoverished areas. In Mississippi, the program came

[45] John Hatch Narrative, *JHC*.

[46] Interview with Dr. Aaron Shirley, Southern Historical Collection, Southern Historical Collection, UNC-Chapel Hill; Paul Francis Howard, S.J., "Report of a Work Project in the Environmental Services Division of Tufts–Delta Health Center, Mound bayou, Mississippi," M.S. Thesis in Environmental Health Engineering, Tufts University, May 1971, located in Box 6, Folder 433a, *DHC,* page 50.

under fire from the state's two U.S. senators, James Eastland and John Stennis, who attacked the Child Development Group of Mississippi (CDGM), which ran the Head Start programs in the state, as being communist and tied to the civil rights movement. In order to appease the powerful senators, who threatened to torpedo much of the War on Poverty agenda, OEO cut off funding to CDGM, and the grant was transferred to another group that was seen as "less threatening to whites in Mississippi," according to Edward Zeigler, who was part of the planning committee for Head Start, and later guided the program as the first director of the Office of Child Development. The first Head Start school in north Bolivar County was eventually opened in Pace, under the auspices of the local health association, in 1970. Another Head Start school was opened in Gunnison, a town of about 800 people by the Mississippi River. That school, which consisted of three mobile classrooms, accommodated 150 preschool children from Gunnison and the surrounding areas.[47]

Indeed, the Head Start program in Mississippi initially had been tied very closely with the civil rights movement, and a number of Tufts–Delta Health Center employees came to work at the health center after working at Head Start. One of them, L. C. Dorsey, recalled, "Many of these community members were drawn to the health center project [had] community organizing experience through civil rights movement activities, or through the War on Poverty program that preceded the health center in Mississippi, Head Start." Given that a number of the health center's organizers, most notably Jack Geiger and Bob Smith, also had been intimately involved in the movement in Mississippi, it is not a surprise that issues of civil, political, and economic rights were often discussed at the health center, and, eventually, at health association meetings. A number of the centers became hubs of political activity, as a newly enfranchised population became cognizant of their potential political power. As Dr. David Weeks, clinical director of the health center, remarked, "People have found out that they can organize and have power, and they have ability."[48]

As a federally funded facility, it was illegal for the Tufts–Delta Health Center to host any type of political events, or have its staff involved in political activities during business hours. The perception by virtually all white Mississippi politicians that the Tufts–Delta Health Center was little more than a front for civil rights

---

[47] Edward Zieger, Sally J. Styfco, and Elizabeth Gilman, "The National Head Start Program for Disadvantaged Preschoolers," in Edward Zieger and Sally J. Styfco, Eds., *Head Start and Beyond* (New Haven and London: Yale University Press, 1993): 1–41; Edward Zeigler and Susan Muenchow, *Head Start* (New York: Basic Books, 1992), ix, 103; Asch, *The Senator & the Sharecropper*, 243–45; Howard, "Report of a Work Project in the Environmental Services Division of Tufts–Delta Health Center," 17, 26–27, 38–40.

[48] Sobelson, "Participation, Power, and Place," 61; McDaniel, "Community Health Centers More Than Clinics for the Poor."

activism, run by communists, put almost all activities run by the center, its employees, the health council, or any of the health associations, under scrutiny from local and state authorities. Nevertheless, center leaders saw the empowerment of the local black community as a central part of their mission in the Delta and did not bow out of their attempts to educate and inspire the people of north Bolivar County to demand their rights. "We would talk to patients about citizen participation, and registering to vote, actually voting after you register—look at the candidates," recalled Dr. Aaron Shirley. "Educating them as to how the system worked, how to take advantage of it."[49]

Because the local health association satellite centers were not owned by Tufts, but were only rented from 7 a.m. to 6 p.m. for health center work, they could be—and were—used for political organizing in the evenings. Many of these meetings were directed by health center staff in connection with local health association leaders, but not during business hours. In order to inspire activism, health center staff engaged in discussions at health association meetings regarding the relationships between raw sewage and poor health; between a substandard diet and ill health; between poor housing and certain diseases; and between poor schools and unemployment. In addition to voter education campaigns, the health associations prepared maps depicting their towns and the distribution of municipal services and facilities, such as sewer lines, fire plugs, paved roads, streetlights, and recreational facilities to illustrate the discrepancies in services between white and black sections of their towns. Health association members also began to attend town meetings and question their local officials, often the first time blacks in any of these towns had attended such meetings. "It was satisfying to see the people themselves assume and support political activism as a pursuit necessary to gaining basic resources important to the quality of life," recalled John Hatch. This political awakening produced real results; within five years, six of the towns in north Bolivar County brought an end to single-race government and succeeded in electing black mayors.[50]

Many of their demands on local governments went unheard, however, and the local health associations also organized a number of boycotts in north Bolivar County to agitate for improved conditions. The first boycott affiliated with the health associations began in May 1968 in Shelby to protest the firing of a principal and a teacher for their work on Kermit Stanton's campaign for the Bolivar County Board of Supervisors. Black elementary and high school students stayed out of class, and there was a boycott of white-owned downtown stores. Headed by L. C. Dorsey,

[49] Interview with Aaron Shirley.
[50] Division of Community Health Action, Progress Reports, 1971 (Box 38, Folder 285), Delta Health Center Papers; John Hatch narrative, *JHC*.

an activist during the civil rights movement who was then employed at the health center, the campaign soon expanded to protest other issues. After Dorsey left work each day she helped organize the protests with members of the Delta Ministry. It was "an example of the total community use of outrage," according to Dorsey. The four-month-long downtown boycott ended when Shelby's city fathers agreed to demands for improved local services, an end to repressive policing, and employment of African Americans by the fire department. The school board refused to rehire the teacher and the principal, but in November Kermit Stanton became the first black elected official in the county since Reconstruction.[51]

Later boycotts centered on the need for improved services in black communities— including sewers, chlorinated water, paved roads, streetlights, recreational facilities, fair treatment by the police, and the employment of blacks in stores, businesses, and municipal agencies, including the police and fire departments. In Rosedale, protests for improved city services were led in the fall of 1970 by Johnny Todd, a local health association member and Tufts–Delta Health Center employee, who would go on to become the town's first black mayor. In Duncan, a boycott of downtown stores began in August 1971 to protest the killing of a black man by a local law enforcement officer. Following the shooting, leaders of the Duncan, Hushpuckena & New Africa Health Association met with city leaders to ask for the removal of the officer, who had shot and paralyzed another black man in Duncan a year earlier. After a series of meetings failed to resolve the issue, health association leaders called for a boycott, and (unsuccessfully) demanded the firing of both the sheriff and the officer.[52]

Political activism by Bolivar County's black population did not go unchallenged. In addition to stonewalling from local officials, the Mississippi State Sovereignty Commission, an internal spy agency established in the 1950s to monitor, infiltrate, and disrupt civil rights activities in the state, also took an interest in the activities in Bolivar County. In particular, Sovereignty Commission officials were obsessed with finding a connection between the Tufts–Delta Health Center and any political activities that would cause it to lose its federal funding. During the Rosedale boycott [see Chapter 4], Sovereignty Commission agents spied on the activities of Tufts employees involved in the protests, and even tried, unsuccessfully, to entice health center employees to become paid informants for the Sovereignty Commission. They

---

[51] Newman, *Divine Agitators*, 169; L. C. Dorsey, *Freedom Came to Mississippi* (New York, N.Y.: The Field Foundation, 1977), 32.

[52] Letter from Rosedale Black Community to Merchants of Rosedale, August 25, 1970 (Series 1, Subseries 1, Box 6, Folder 44) *DHC*; The Duncan, Hushpuckena and New Africa Health Association, Progress Report, 1971 (Box 38, Folder 285), *DHC*; Owen Taylor, "Duncan Invisible Boycott," *Delta Democrat-Times*, September 5, 1971.

were eventually frustrated in their inability to make any direct link between the health center leadership and the boycott.[53]

* * *

Although improved health care was the main focus of the Tufts–Delta Health Center, community activism was always another major goal of the founders of the center. Born of the idealism—and frustration—of the civil rights movement in Mississippi, the health center sought to serve as a catalyst for the dispossessed peoples of the Delta to empower themselves. Central to providing the people of north Bolivar County more control over their quality of life was the creation of the ten health associations and the North Bolivar County Health Council. It was these associations, built from the ground up, that gave the poor people of the area a say—often for the very first time—in decisions that affected their children, their homes, their neighborhoods, and their towns. "Community organizing is probably the most important thing done in the center," Andy James stated. "It has turned things on for some small towns."[54] The economic and educational opportunities that the health center provided were also critical to improving the lives of many people of the Delta. With its federal funding, the health center provided jobs for the unemployed in one of the poorest parts of the nation, providing what amounted to direct work relief, which not only improved the conditions of those with jobs at the health center, but also impacted the economy of the wider community. More lasting were the careers that began as a result of both the occupational and educational opportunities provided by the health center and its partners. "I think in any oppressed society you are going to find some brilliant folk, who are of genius level, who just never had an opportunity to express it," remarked John Hatch. "When you provide a pathway, a lot of people who are gonna do it. There were many people . . . who through various programs at the health center, found that pathway . . ., [they] just needed the tiniest bit of opportunity to make a much better life."[55] Finally, the center helped cultivate a new generation of indigenous leaders in the Delta. Many of those who were able to acquire an education and develop a career through the intervention of the Tufts–Delta Health Center's staff eventually returned to Mississippi.

---

[53] James M. Mohead, "Weekly Reports [SCR ID # 99-1-0-12-1-1-1 and 99-1-0-14-1-1-1], Mississippi Sovereignty Commission files, Mississippi Department of Archives and History, Sovereignty Commission Online (http://mdah.state.ms.us/arrec/digital_archives/sovcom/), hereafter *MSC*.

[54] McDaniel, "Community Health Centers More Than Clinics for the Poor."

[55] Ward interview with John Hatch and Jack Geiger.

To treat symptoms, and then to send patients back, unchanged in knowledge, attitude
or behavior, to the same physical and social environment—also unchanged—that
overwhelmingly helped produce their illness and will do so again, is to provide antibiotics for
cholera and then send patients back to drink again from the Broad Street pump.

H. JACK GEIGER

3

Delivering Health Care

BOTH THE TRIUMPHS and scars of the civil rights movement were still fresh in Mississippi when Tufts's temporary health clinic opened in November 1967 in a five-room church parsonage, just off Route 61 in Mound Bayou. Jack Geiger recalled that "[we used] the living room as a waiting room, [several] bedroom[s] as . . . examining room[s], and a kitchen for a laboratory, and said 'we are open'." Along with the church parsonage, the Tufts team remodeled an abandoned storefront into a prenatal care unit, used an old theater as a school to train locals to be health aides, and brought in a trailer to serve as the business office. On opening day they saw only eight people, as there was still a great deal of skepticism about the center. "People did what they always do, they sent scouts to see what it was about," remembered Geiger, but "by the end of the week the word was out and there were a hundred people trying to come through the place."[1]

The center's initial staff consisted of Jack Geiger and John Hatch, five registered nurses, a social worker, and three Northern white physicians—Leon Kruger, Christian Hansen, and Roy Brown—who all received appointments on the Tufts Medical School faculty after agreeing to move with their families to Mississippi to take part in the Mound Bayou health center project. Kruger, the center's first clinical

---

[1] Interview with H. Jack Geiger by Robert Korstad and Neil Boothby; "Medicine: Treating the Poor," *Time*, Nov. 29, 1968.

director, gave up a thriving practice in the wealthy Boston suburb of Newton to come to Mound Bayou, while Brown was a New York pediatrician who previously had served at the Columbia Point Health Center. Hansen was a Pennsylvania native and member of the Medical Committee for Human Rights who also had worked with Jack Geiger and Count Gibson in Boston. Dr. Robert Smith approached Hansen about joining the health center during a trip to Mississippi. "Bob told me about a plan for building a comprehensive rural health center in Mound Bayou," recalled Hansen. "He wondered if I would like to be a part of the project, too." Hansen was intrigued. "The prospect of working in Mound Bayou and opening a health center there appealed to me tremendously. A dozen years of training—medical school, residency, working on reservations, training Peace Corps volunteers, then public health school—now seemed like a prologue. This, finally, was something I wanted to do."[2]

Smith and Dr. Aaron Shirley, a fellow Mississippian, also joined the health center's staff on a part-time basis, each commuting the 130 miles to Mound Bayou one or two days a week from their homes and practices in Jackson. Shirley would leave home at six a.m., drive to Mound Bayou, then return to Jackson in the evening, while Smith took flying lessons so he could pilot himself in a borrowed plane back and forth to the Delta. "I'd get up at 4 o'clock in the morning and make rounds, be at the Jackson airport at, oh, 7.30, and [then] I'd be landing in Mound Bayou," he recalled. "I'd do that once a week."[3]

Bob Smith, a stout, powerfully built man, was born in 1937 in Terry, Mississippi, just south of Jackson, the ninth of twelve children. His father was a livestock dealer and a farmer; his grandfather had been a sharecropper. Smith attended the all-black school in Terry, where four teachers taught all eight grades. He was influenced to pursue medicine by an elderly Jewish physician who hunted with his father and gave the younger Smith his medical books when he retired. "He brought those medical books home, and I started thumbing through those books," Smith recalled, "and that captured my real imagination." Smith attended Tougaloo College in Jackson, then Howard Medical School in Washington, DC, because the University of Mississippi Medical School did not then admit blacks. He received $5,000 in loans from the state to attend medical school as part of the Mississippi Medical Education Program, loans that would be forgiven if he returned to Mississippi and practiced in the state for five years. This program was instituted to preserve segregation by providing an opportunity for black Mississippians to attend medical school

[2] Hall, "A Stir of Hope in Mound Bayou," 70; Dittmer, *The Good Doctors*, 232; Christian M. Hansen, *In the Name of the Children: The Life Story of a Pediatrician to the Poor* (Ipswich, Mass.: Roger Warner, 2005), 52.
[3] Dittmer, *The Good Doctors*, 232; Interview with Dr. Robert Smith by Tom Ward, Cleveland, Mississippi, June 8, 2013.

without integrating the University of Mississippi Medical School. This situation troubled Smith, but he reasoned that: "If I hadn't taken it, I wouldn't be a doctor today."[4]

While at Howard, Smith first met Martin Luther King Jr., and when he returned to Mississippi in 1962 to start his medical career, the civil rights movement was beginning to gain steam. Smith took a position at a state hospital for the mentally ill, and also began providing free medical services for students at Tougaloo, a haven for civil rights activists, whom Smith treated for free, eventually earning him the moniker, "doctor to the movement." His civil rights activities cost him his state job, so he opened up a private practice in Jackson and continued his work with the movement, establishing himself as a leader in the Medical Committee for Human Rights, where he became close with Jack Geiger, and served as Martin Luther King's personal physician during the 1966 March Against Fear through Mississippi. "I marched side by side with him down the road," Smith recalled. "I just knew Martin Luther King was going to be assassinated."[5]

Like Bob Smith, Aaron Shirley was born and raised in segregated Mississippi and educated at Tougaloo. The youngest of eight children, Shirley was reared in Jackson by his mother, a nurse's aide, after his father died when Shirley was an infant. As had Smith, Shirley took advantage of Mississippi's Medical Education Program and enrolled at Meharry Medical College in Nashville, which, along with Howard, trained the vast majority of the nation's black physicians during the Jim Crow era. After completing an internship he returned to Mississippi in 1960 to work off his tuition obligation with the state. He settled in Vicksburg when the town's only black physician was retiring, but found that segregation limited his opportunities to treat patients. "No black doctor had . . . [hospital] privileges in Vicksburg," Shirley recalled. "I was delivering babies in my office. It soon became obvious I couldn't fulfill my obligations without breaking some barriers." He took the issue of discrimination at the hospital to the U.S. Justice Department, but it was not until 1965, two months before he left the city, that he was finally invited to join the hospital staff.[6]

Like Bob Smith, Aaron Shirley's civil rights activism soon extended beyond medical issues. Along with his wife, Ollye, Shirley became increasing involved with the movement as it centered on Mississippi, engaging in voting rights activities and even founding a newspaper to report on African-American issues, with Ollye serving as editor. Unable to get the paper printed in Mississippi, they sent it to New Orleans

[4] Dittmer, *The Good Doctors*, 1–3; 8; "An interview with Robert Smith, M.D." by Harriet Tanzman; Ward, *Black Physicians in the Jim Crow South*, 43.

[5] Dittmer, *The Good Doctors*, 8–9, 14, 16, 23–24, 154.

[6] Dittmer, *The Good Doctors*, 25–27; Lefkowitz, *Community Health Centers*. 32–33.

for publication. When approached by Jack Geiger to get involved with the development of the health center, Shirley jumped at the opportunity. "Having been a part of the movement, this was just another extension of what we've been doing already," he remembered. "And the concept, to me, was something totally new, but it was exciting—empowering people."[7]

* * *

In their planning of the health center, Geiger and Gibson had focused on the dramatic needs of infants and children in the Delta. They knew of the high infant mortality rates in the region: The black infant mortality rate in Bolivar County in 1964 was 56.2 per 1,000 live births, twice the rate for all of Mississippi, which had the worst infant mortality rate in the nation. They therefore believed that much of the health center's focus would be on pediatric care. As a result, they recruited pediatricians like Kruger, Hansen, and Brown to come to Mound Bayou. What the first weeks and months of the clinic's opening showed them was that—although the need for children's health services was indeed acute—there was also a tremendous demand for a host of adult health services that they had not anticipated, such as treating hypertension and arthritis. "When we first came here, we thought we would be overwhelmed with kids," Geiger recalled. "But we got whomped with older people with chronic illnesses who had been sitting out there unattended." Aura Kruger remembered finding her husband, who expected to be treating children when he came to Mississippi, sitting at the dining room table each morning "with his old medical books, reading everything he could about diseases of the elderly," while Chris Hansen remembered being "deluged with adults who had aches and pains, and colorful expressions for their ailments. The patients called diabetes 'sugar.' Anemia was 'low blood' and hypertension was 'high blood.'" Additionally, he recalled, because "many of the older adults we saw had chronic health problems such as back pain from years of leaning over to pick cotton . . . [we tried] to do a complete medical history and a physical exam" of each of them.[8]

Within a few weeks of opening its doors, the clinic was seeing as many as a hundred people a day, and by the spring of 1968 demands on the center's services forced it to move out of the small parsonage and into an intermediate facility (a series of prefabricated buildings set up on the grounds purchased for the center) while the permanent structure was being completed. The demand on the center contradicted

[7] Lefkowitz, *Community Health Centers*, 32–33; Interview with Dr. Aaron Shirley by Dr. John Hatch (July 18, 1992), Southern Historical Collection, UNC–Chapel Hill.

[8] Neil Maxwell, "The Ailing Poor," *Wall Street Journal* (Jan. 14, 1969); Christian Hansen, "The Pediatrician and Family Planning in a Very Poor Community: An Appraisal of Experiences in the Tufts Delta Health Ctr., Bolivar County, Mississippi." *Clinical Pediatrics* (June 1972): 319–23; Ivester, *The Outskirts of Hope*, 66; Hansen, *In the Name of the Children*, 63, 65.

the earlier protests by white Mississippi politicians and physicians that the center was unnecessary because the black poor of the Delta received adequate care. The rural poor were, indeed, willing to come from their small towns and hamlets across the county to the Tufts–Delta Health Center because it offered thorough examinations, accurate diagnosis, and effective treatment, in contrast to the indifference and disrespect often shown toward poor people by doctors—both black and white—at the fraternal hospitals and in private practice.[9]

The intermediate facility was a great improvement over the parsonage; it was air-conditioned and had fifteen rooms. It sat on twenty acres of land Tufts agreed to purchase from a local black farmer using part of its federal grant. When it came time to build the permanent center, however, there were some significant difficulties. In order to build the center, John Hatch had obtained an option on the land from its owner, Mr. Latham, to secure the purchase, pending Office of Economic Opportunity (OEO) approval. As a goodwill gesture, he had then given the option plus a $100 fee to the Mound Bayou Development Corporation for it to hold until the purchase was ready to be completed. Later, when the sale was approved by the federal government, the Mound Bayou Development Corporation refused to turn over the option except on the condition that it owned the land and ran the health center, which was totally unacceptable to Tufts and OEO. Geiger recalled that, "when it became clear that there were no other ways around it, I called a meeting of all of the staff [and] . . . I said if this didn't get resolved we would simply have to go elsewhere and that we could do that." If Tufts removed the health center from Mound Bayou at that point, when over fifty people from across the county had already been hired, and about fifty more were expecting jobs, it would have been devastating to the local economy. Mr. Latham, who owned the land, went to meet the board members of the development corporation—carrying his shotgun with him—explaining that he did not see what the problem was. It was his land and Tufts's money, so what did they have to do with it? Eventually, an agreement was reached when the development corporation returned the option to Mr. Latham and the land sale was concluded.[10]

The problems in constructing the permanent structure did not end there. The original law that created OEO prohibited the use of War on Poverty funds to be used to build any "brick and mortar" structures, so the Tufts team initially looked for an acceptable building to renovate, which was permissible under federal guidelines, without success. Geiger then advocated purchasing prefabricated units,

[9] Hall, "A Stir of Hope in Mound Bayou," 70; DeJong, "Plantation Politics," 262.

[10] Hall, "A Stir of Hope in Mound Bayou," 70; Interview with Jack Geiger by Korstad and Boothby.

which did not seem to violate the OEO's prohibition on construction. He contacted a company in California that produced modular buildings and arranged to have them shipped to Mississippi. The units—sixty feet by twenty feet—started to arrive in Mound Bayou in the spring of 1968. The company sent its own crew to put the units together on the foundation and complete the plumbing and wiring. Geiger remembered that an all-black crew came from Los Angeles to do the work. One morning they came to him and asked that he hire guards for the project. "We said, 'Why?'" Geiger recalled. "They said that somebody local—we later learned it was one of those [local black] physicians—came and offered us $5,000 to blow it all up. [The health center] was seen as a competitive threat."[11]

Despite all these obstacles, in December 1968 the health center staff—which by that time numbered 120, one hundred of whom were local black residents of Bolivar County who had been trained and hired to work at the center—moved into their $900,000, state-of-the-art, 24,000-square-foot clinic building in Mound Bayou. The facility was equipped with consulting rooms, examining rooms, an emergency room, an X-ray unit, a clinical laboratory, and a complete pharmacy, as well as waiting rooms for patients and conference rooms for staff training and staff meetings. It also had office facilities for the Environmental Services Unit, the North Bolivar County Health Council, the Community Health Action, Community Organizing and Health Education Unit, the Clinical Director, the Medical Librarian, the social workers, and other staff. Although the delay in moving into a permanent structure was difficult, in retrospect Geiger saw it as a blessing, because it allowed his team to focus on community organizing, hiring and training health center staff, conducting a census and health survey of the black residents of north Bolivar County, and engaging in community outreach. "It was during this period that people began to raise issues beyond medical care," he recalled.[12]

Much of the interest in the health center (and demand for its services) was attributable to the work on the ground by John Hatch. As he had when scouting locations in the Delta for the health center the year before, once the center opened Hatch and his team spent much of their time out in the community garnering support and identifying needs. One of Hatch's goals was to counter the continuing suspicion the center faced. "We found distrust was pervasive," he recalled. "Those whose income, power or prestige might be threatened by our project would probably oppose us. . . . Gatekeeper blacks were concerned about the implications of an operation . . .

[11] Interview with Jack Geiger by Korstad and Boothby.

[12] Assorted notes on construction, Series 1, Subseries 1, Box 1, Folder 5 DHC; Hall, "A Stir of Hope in Mound Bayou," 69; "Medicine: Treating the Poor," Time Nov. 29, 1968; Sobelson, "Participation, Power, and Place," 64–65.

functioning outside their sphere of control . . ., militant blacks questioned the appropriateness of a 'white' institution . . . in a predominantly black community; others felt that all such programs amounted to pacification." Undeterred, Hatch engaged in dialogues throughout the county, encouraging people to come to the health center and make use of its services. Although he emphasized that, "We certainly could not assure each of these varied groups that the center would always operate within a framework acceptable to them . . . once we recruited a local staff of 12 and clinical services began, our credibility greatly increased."[13]

Another difficulty the center faced in attracting patients was what Roy Brown described as "a significant cultural gap between [the] professional and [the] consumer," which he compared to practicing medicine in developing countries. Even with a free and accessible medical facility, and a comprehensive approach to health care, there were often difficulties in getting people the care they needed, none more significant than an unwillingness to seek care. "What may be considered by the staff as 'illness,'" he wrote, "often is accepted by the rural population as a permissible deviation from 'full health,'" and medical attention is not sought. Getting patients the care they needed was not as simple as just the creation of a health facility, with the expectation that those in need would come to their doors; the doctors and nurses also needed to learn how to communicate in a new way in order to define sickness and health for their patients. "It is necessary for health professionals to assume a far greater responsibility among extremely poor rural families," argued Brown, "than [just] the strict diagnosis and treatment of presenting acute illness."[14]

Geiger always had intended to create a comprehensive health center that focused on much more than just the types of basic services that one would find at a county health department, but he and his team initially were not prepared to deal with the wants and needs of his target population. In addition to communication problems and the large number of geriatric issues, the Tufts team also soon found that many of the services that they hoped to provide were not necessarily desired by members of the community—some were even resented—while there were significant needs that they had not anticipated. As Hatch traveled throughout the county promoting the center, he found that discussions of improved maternal and child care—a priority of the center—often were met with resistance from mothers, who frequently regarded such discussions as indictments of their ability to raise their children properly. The common use of home remedies, roots, and even faith healers in the Mississippi Delta

---

[13] Larry T. Patton, "Community Health Centers: The Early Years of the Movement," (unpublished manuscript), *JGC*; Hall, "A Stir of Hope in Mound Bayou," 73.

[14] Roy E. Brown, "Delivery of Pediatric Health Services in A Rural Health Center," *Pediatrics* Vol. 44, No. 3 (September, 1969): 333–37.

was another area of contention. "Residents of Bolivar County were well aware that practitioners of scientific medicine usually question the propriety of remedies," wrote Hatch, "and [they] were no more willing to share information that presented the possibility of causing ridicule or censure than most of us." Before they could deliver health care, the Tufts staff needed to be able to communicate effectively and build trust with those whom they sought to serve.[15]

The single most important discovery by the Tufts staff was the rampant malnutrition within the community. Geiger recalled that only about two weeks after opening the clinic, he met with some of the locals who had come to the center. "How are we doing and what do you think of the health service?" he asked. They said, "Oh, the health service and the doctors I saw in there were just fine, but you know, we think we would be healthier if you had something to eat—can you do something about food?" Other members of the Tufts' staff had similar experiences, and, as Hatch later wrote, "We soon found out that the number one priority was not health as traditionally viewed. Food, that is the lack of it, was the most pressing problem in the fall and winter of 1967. . . . Existing programs aimed toward avoiding malnutrition were not working."[16]

The public health nurses who made home visits regularly observed that people often had little more than some grits and beans in their home, while some residents shot squirrels and gathered pecans to supplement their families' diets. The center's physicians regularly saw the effects of malnutrition in those who came to the clinic for care. One observer wrote that, "These children in Mississippi live on a diet of cornbread, grits, and Kool-aid," and "the effects of malnutrition are staggering. . . . Skin disease is rampant with . . . children suffering from rashes, boils, dryness and shrinkage" as "prolonged protein deficiency in some children has caused the body to consume its own protein tissue." The malnutrition crisis that ravaged the black residents of the Delta was especially acute for infants, because, as Leon Kruger stated, "malnutrition in the first year is irreversible," in its effects on a child's development.[17] Christian Hansen recalled an infant who was brought to the clinic early in his tenure:

---

[15] North Bolivar County farm cooperative self-help nutritional program. Grant proposal (written by John Hatch), 1972, *JHC*; North Bolivar County farm cooperative self-help nutritional program. Grant proposal (written by John Hatch), 1972, *JHC*.

[16] Interview with H. Jack Geiger by Robert Korstad and Neil Boothby; John Hatch, "Community Development in a Rural Comprehensive Community Health Program," paper presented at the New York Academy of Medicine annual health conference, April 24, 1970, *JHC*.

[17] Herbert Black, *People and Plows Against Hunger: Self-Help Experiment in a Rural Community* (Boston: Marlborough House, Inc., 1975), 4.; "Where Everything's Fine," St. Louis *Post-Dispatch*, March 30, 1968.

Aaron Shirley and I examined a month-old baby boy who was suffering from severe malnutrition. When we first saw the baby, I didn't think he was going to live. His gasping breath, the listless rolling of the eyes, and his weak cry were all too familiar signs of impending death. I took a closer look. In addition to the malnutrition, he was severely dehydrated. . . . The baby's skin hung like dried folds over his stomach, and his mouth was parched. His eyes were so dry there were no tears when he cried. His arms and legs were lacking in both fatty and muscle tissue. . . .

One of the nurses cradled the baby in her arms and I shaved his head, trying to find a vein large enough to insert an intravenous needle. . . . Meanwhile, Dr. Shirley placed a small oxygen mask over the baby's nose and mouth, and covered him with blankets to prevent him from going into shock. . . .

The mother had originally brought [the baby] to a doctor who saw as many as 200 patients a day [in Shelby]. He told her to stop milk for two days and feed him water and "pot likker"—the broth left in the pot after vegetables had been cooked, which is filled with vitamins, but is only a supplementary food. It was good advice, but she needed to start feeding the child after two days, which she failed to do. By the time the baby came to the center he weighed less than he had at birth. The baby died.[18]

Aaron Shirley later angrily recounted this incident to a newspaper reporter, who asked why such a thing was able to happen. "Ignorance and poverty," Shirley replied bluntly, "and one breeds the other."[19]

To combat the malnutrition crisis they found, Geiger and Hatch came up with an innovative solution, one that caused a great deal of controversy with both their federal funders and the Mississippi governor once they found out about it: The center's physicians began to write prescriptions for food. "We decided that wherever we saw [malnourished] children . . . we would provide them with food: so much milk, so much eggs, so much meat, so much vegetables. We'd do it by writing them a prescription for food," said Geiger. A deal was made with one, then eventually ten, grocery stores in black communities in northern Bolivar County to fill the food prescriptions and send the bill to the Tufts–Delta Health Center for reimbursement, which the health center paid for out of its pharmacy budget. It was a radical idea that Geiger had taken from his experience in South Africa, where Sidney Kark had provided dried skim milk to starving children, classifying it as a medicine. When

---

[18] Hansen, *In the Name of the Children*, 66–69.
[19] Richard Lyons, "Grip of Poverty Chokes Mississippi Children," Memphis *Commercial Appeal* (April 1, 1968).

OEO got word that Geiger was buying food out of his pharmacy budget, it was incredulous. Geiger recalled his conversation with an OEO official: "[They said,] 'How could you do this, what do you think you're doing, you can't use a pharmacy for that!' I said, 'Why not?' They said, 'Because a pharmacy is for drugs, for the treatment of disease'. And I said, 'That's right, and the last time we looked in the book for specific therapy for malnutrition, it was food'. They went away because there was nothing they could say to something that stupid but that true!" As another physician at the center noted, "If mothers and babies don't eat, all the medicine in the world won't work."[20]

The malnutrition crisis in Mississippi's Delta region was a product of both extreme poverty and failed government policy and procedures. The War on Poverty created food stamps, which replaced the commodities program that had previously distributed free staples like flour, powdered milk, canned goods, and eggs to the poor. The food stamp program, however, required recipients to first document their poverty to prove their eligibility, and then pay hard cash to get the stamps, which could then be redeemed at stores for groceries. For example, it cost a family of six about $12 a month for food stamps, even if it had no income at all, which meant that many poor in the Delta lost the food commodities they had relied on for survival, but could not afford food stamps. A reporter from Wisconsin found in a tour of the Mississippi Delta that "people are being taken off welfare and [the costs of] food stamps are being raised. We met a mother of four who must pay $52 for $82 worth of food stamps. Her welfare check has been reduced to $30 a month because she works as a janitoress at a local grade school." In 1967, the *Boston Globe* provided a harsh assessment of the distribution of federal funds for the poor in Mississippi, reporting that, "The tragedy of stark, prolonged poverty turns to terror in Mississippi where the welfare system is an extension of the white power structure and does not reach thousands of families. Public welfare in Bolivar County and all areas of Mississippi is a function of the county board of supervisors. In Bolivar County, white men decide who will get aid and how much."[21]

Because of these failures, the center continued with its "food prescription" program, extending it to include baby formula and eventually having the program written—appropriately—into the center's OEO budget. "We had to write up [to Washington] and say, 'Look, we are now going to have to write up prescriptions for

---

[20] Kark and Kark, *Promoting Community Health*, 49; Interview with H. Jack Geiger by Robert Korstad and Neil Boothby; Lefkowitz, *Community Health Center*, 38.

[21] Dittmer, *The Good Doctors*, 232–33; Cobb, *The Most Southern Place on Earth*, 259–60; "My First Trip to Ole Miss," *Madison* (Wisconsin) *Sun*, October 26, 1968; "Tufts Plan: Negroes' Only Ray of Hope," *Boston Globe*, July 16, 1967.

Carnation milk and evaporated milk so we can teach these mothers how to make milk to feed their babies,' " recalled Dr. Helen Barnes, the health center's director of obstetrics and gynecology. "So [OEO] allowed us to reshuffle money that they had designated for something else, X number of thousands of dollars . . . [and] when the pregnancy got to 38 weeks I would start writing prescriptions for Carnation milk or evaporated milk." In 1970, Greenville, Mississippi's *Delta Democrat-Times* reported that OEO approved a $68,731 grant for an emergency food and medical services project to the Tufts–Delta Health Center and the Mound Bayou Community Hospital, which would be administered by the North Bolivar County Health Council. The funds were to be used "to improve the diets of pregnant mothers, infants, and children up to 6 years old in low-income families. The program includes a unique 'food prescription' proposal which will enable doctors to prescribe certain foods for patients. The prescriptions will be filled at one of seven food distribution centers to be opened in Bolivar County." The paper also reported that approximately 5,000 people had registered for the program.[22]

Malnutrition contributed greatly to almost all the other ailments of Bolivar County's poor. Thelma Walker, the head nurse at Tufts–Delta Health Center, recalled a case where a nurse paying a routine call on an elderly man with hypertension and his severely disabled daughter found that there was absolutely no food in the house. The nurse filled out a "food prescription" for chicken, ground beef, potatoes, shortening, coffee, milk, cornmeal, and other staples to be provided by the center. Dr. Florence Halpern, the health center's psychologist, found that the deprived diets of the area's children had depressed their development, perhaps permanently. Meanwhile, Geiger fought to try to solve the problem of what he deemed marasmus—the wasting away of the body due to inadequate food. In addition to the lack of food, the diets of many poor blacks in the Delta contributed to a host of ailments. High blood pressure was a common problem among the center's target population, but salt pork, which greatly aggravated the condition, was a staple found in most black homes in the region. Consumption of some of the other foods that were most readily available—potatoes, beans, and grits—even had the result of making someone overweight but still malnourished. Nurses and nutritionists worked with the local population to try and improve diets, but both poverty and culture often stood in their way. Estelle Rodriguez, a nursing administrator at the health center, explained how she worked to get people to make small changes that could help improve their health: "I show her how to trim the fat off, how to lift the greens up out

---

[22] Interview with Dr. Helen Barns by Tom Ward, August 25, 2015; "OEO Grant Set for Mound Bayou," *Delta Democrat-Times* (Greenville, Miss.), July 5, 1970.

of the fat instead of dishing them out, swimming in fat. This doesn't make her diet letter perfect, but at least it reduces the cholesterol and the salt."[23]

* * *

When the Tufts–Delta Health Center opened the doors of its permanent facility in late 1968, it was able to provide a wide variety of services on-site, with examination and consulting rooms, an emergency room, pharmacy, laboratory, X-ray, social work, and clinical nursing services all available. By 1970, the center was averaging 2,500 patient visits a month, providing everything from basic immunizations for children to mental health care administered by an in-house clinical psychologist. The center was not designed, however, to provide any type of hospital care. Instead, the health center engaged in an important, but often difficult, partnership with the Mound Bayou Community Hospital.[24]

When Geiger and Hatch scouted Mound Bayou as a possible location for the health center, the presence of not one, but two, black-owned and run hospitals in the small town intrigued them greatly, because they saw the possibilities for very promising collaborations between the health center and the hospitals. These hospitals, the Taborian and the Sarah Brown, were both private, for-profit enterprises, owned and run by fraternal organizations. By the mid-1960s, each was in dire financial straits and deteriorating structurally. Geiger understood the value of a hospital in close proximity to the proposed health center, and he helped negotiate a separate OEO grant to the two hospitals in 1966, with the provision that they be united into a community hospital, and no longer limit their clientele to dues-paying members of the fraternal organizations. As a result, in 1967 the Mound Bayou Community Hospital was organized to unify the services of the two facilities. The OEO provided $1 million to modernize, equip, and staff the old Taborian Hospital as the new Mound Bayou Community Hospital, and to convert the Sarah Brown Hospital into a dental clinic. The renovated facility had a more modern operating room, labor and delivery suites, new beds, and more full-time nursing staff. As part of the grant agreement, all physicians from the Tufts–Delta Health Center also would be granted visiting staff privileges at the hospital.[25]

In addition to the unification of the fraternal hospitals, Meharry Medical College in Nashville, one of the nation's two surviving historically black medical schools,

[23] Maxwell, "The Ailing Poor"; "Where Everything's Fine," St. Louis *Post-Dispatch*, March 30, 1968; Cynthia Kelly, "Health Care in the Mississippi Delta," 763; Richard Knox, "Hope Comes to Mound Bayou," *Boston Globe* (April 26, 1970).

[24] C. G. McDaniel, "Community Health Centers More Than Clinics for the Poor"; DeJong, "Plantation Politics," 262.

[25] "Moral Consciousness and Commitment in Mound Bayou," *Meharry Medical College Quarterly Digest* (January 1970), 11–15; "New Hospital is First Tangible By-Product of Tufts Project" *Boston Globe*, July 18, 1967.

which had a long association with Taborian Hospital, also received an OEO grant to both continue its work in Mound Bayou and to establish a community health center in Nashville. The grant was written in large part by Geiger and Count Gibson, in collaboration with faculty and administrators from Meharry, and was part of an effort to smooth relationships with Meharry, which understandably felt it had been ignored and displaced by the Tufts project. This grant also provided funding for a department of community medicine at Meharry.[26]

The relationship between Taborian Hospital and Meharry Medical College went back to the year the hospital opened, when its directors approached Dr. Matthew Walker, then an assistant professor of surgery and gynecology at Meharry, to become the chief surgeon at Taborian. Walker, a Louisiana native and Meharry graduate, was one of the first African Americans to become a fellow of the American College of Surgeons. He declined the position in Mound Bayou, choosing instead to stay at his alma mater. He again was approached by the directors of Taborian in 1947 when its chief of surgery left, but Walker again declined the post. This time, however, he proposed a program that he believed would benefit both the patients of Taborian Hospital and the students of Meharry. Walker suggested that he provide Taborian with surgical residents from Meharry on a rotating basis. This plan sought to alleviate Meharry's problem of finding available spots for its graduates to serve residencies, given that black physicians were barred from practicing at most hospitals in the South at the time, as well as Taborian's problem of maintaining a well-trained staff at a price it could afford. The plan called for Meharry to send two residents to serve four- to six-month stints in Mound Bayou as the hospital's chief surgeon and assistant. Walker also periodically made the 200-mile trip from Nashville to check on his charges and to perform any difficult or risky operations better not left to the residents.[27]

Despite some difficulties, the health center and the hospital found many ways to work together to improve the health of the Delta's impoverished population. Viola Chandler, the director of nursing at the hospital, recruited Thelma Walker, the nursing administrator of the health center, to coordinate nursing care from rural areas of the county to the center or the hospital and back to the community. The two women also developed service programs for their staffs, and instituted

---

[26] Jack Geiger notes, *JGC*.

[27] Ward, *Black Physicians in the Jim Crow South*, 70–71; Meharry Medical College Press Release (July 17, 1978), Folder 6, Box 1, Matthew Walker Papers, Meharry Medical College Archives, Nashville, Tenn.; Matthew Walker, "The Affiliation of Taborian Hospital with Meharry Medical College and Development of the OEO Planning Grant," 3; James Summerville, *Educating Black Doctors: A History of Meharry Medical College*, (Tuscaloosa, Ala.: University of Alabama Press, 1983), 92–95.

a rotation program, so that nurses from both the hospital and the health center were familiar with one another's facilities and practices. For example, health center nurses went on assignment at the hospital to refresh their knowledge of acute care, while hospital staff nurses worked in the center to learn about its outreach programs and clinics.[28]

Because they had admitting privileges at the hospital, the health center's physicians could provide their patients emergency services and other care that the Tufts–Delta Health Center was not equipped to handle. Christian Hansen recalled one instance in which, "Since our clinic had only outpatient facilities, I carried Otis [who had meningitis] across the road to the community hospital. . . . We were able to save Otis, and eventually he recovered without brain damage." In addition to the Mound Bayou Community Hospital, the Tufts–Delta Health Center also worked with other hospitals in the region. Some health center doctors used the small, private hospital in Shelby, ten miles from Mound Bayou, to hospitalize their patients, paying the white doctor who ran it for his services. For more serious hospital needs, however, it was necessary to transport patients to Memphis (100 miles away) or Jackson (150 miles away). The East Bolivar County Hospital, only fourteen miles away in Cleveland, was a large, modern, facility that could have saved patients some of the long trips to Memphis and Jackson, but it required a $50 cash deposit for admitting any uninsured patients, did not accept uninsured patients whose bills were paid for by OEO, and did not offer admitting privileges to the health center's physicians.[29]

Much of the care provided by the Tufts–Delta Health Center was not delivered at either the center or the hospital. As Geiger recalled, "A lot of the people we took care of we took care of in their own shacks."[30] Nurses like Thelma Walker and Estelle Rodriguez left Mound Bayou daily to take to the roads of Bolivar County to visit those in need, often covering 100 to 150 miles a day. One of the nurses described her typical day:

> After I get all my materials together, I leave about 9:30, sometimes 10 o'clock—this is after I've checked with the doctors concerning their patients. Getting the equipment out . . . carrying pads, perhaps wheelchairs provided to some of the patients, carrying the medications. . . . I usually have certain days that I see certain patients. I see from five to six patients a day, sometimes four, it depends on the condition of the patient. I spend from 15 minutes to

[28] Kelly, "Health Care in in the Mississippi Delta," 762.

[29] Hansen, *In the Name of the Children*, 66; Howard, "Report of a Work Project in the Environmental Services Division of Tufts–Delta Health Center."

[30] Geiger interview with Ward.

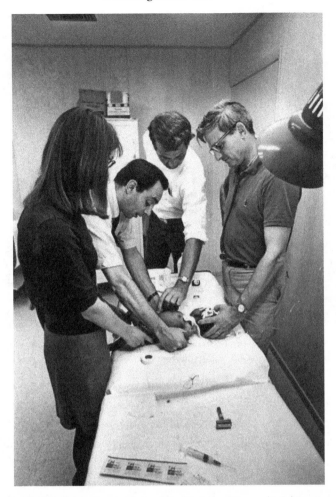

FIGURE 3.1 Dr. H. Jack Geiger (leaning in) and Dr. Christian Hansen (right) treating a dehydrated baby at the Tufts–Delta Health Center (Photo courtesy of Dan Bernstein, Southern Historical Collection, University of North Carolina at Chapel Hill).

sometimes three hours with the patient in the home, teaching and instructing [such as how to take care for a sick child, how to administer medicine, etc.], and assisting them with their needs. . . .

My first patient every day . . . has had a stroke, she's bedridden. I go there in the morning, I assist her stepdaughter. . . . We have to do everything for her, including feed her, and she usually pulls her catheter out, we have to reinsert it, if the doctor wants us to—we have to check with him first. I provide routine nursing care, routine nursing procedures, in the home, and instructions, advice to the different members of the family.[31]

---

[31] Mrs. White Oral History, Delta Health Center Tapes, Disk 1, Reel 5–9.

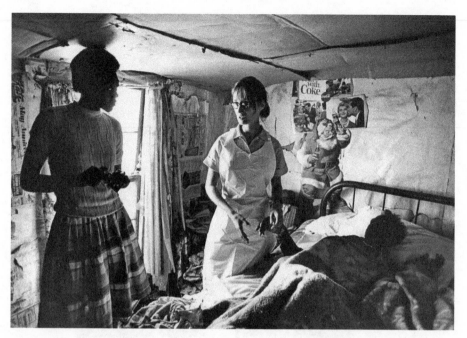

FIGURE 3.2   A Tufts–Delta Health Center nurse making a home visit (Photo courtesy of Dan Bernstein, Southern Historical Collection, University of North Carolina at Chapel Hill).

A whole team of traveling health center nurses routinely made upwards of 300 visits a week throughout the 500-square-mile area of northern Bolivar County served by the health center, providing a wide variety of services for those unable to get to Mound Bayou. Finding the homes was sometimes an adventure in itself, because patients often lived in plantation shacks, unmarked with any address or name. Nurses often relied on hand-drawn maps, with directions such as "[go] three hickory tree down the road, then turn right at the dead tree." Often they resorted to knocking on doors to ask if anyone knew the person they were looking for and where they lived. Once someone's home was located, the nurse wrote down directions, or even made her own hand-drawn map, and attached it to the patient's chart.[32]

Thelma Walker stated that simply getting to the poor and scattered population in a rural area was the most significant difference from her previous nursing experiences, because "dogs, dust in summer or mud in winter, and distances slow us down." The dirt roads of rural Bolivar County were sometimes impassable when the rains came and turned them to mud, or were full of deep ruts when baked by the Mississippi sun. Flat tires were a regular occurrence, and the nurses often had

---

[32] Sister Mary Stella Simpson, *Sister Stella's Babies* (New York: American Journal of Nursing Company Educational Services Division, 1978), 28, 35; Kelly, "Health Care in the Mississippi Delta," 759–60.

to park far from the patient's home and walk to the house, carrying all their equipment with them, in order to save their vehicles. Walker also said that in the Delta
she saw more mothers with toxemia and eclampsia; more children with rheumatic
fever and diarrhea; more people of all ages with iron deficiency anemia; and more
elderly persons with ankylosed joints followed by cerebrovascular accidents, than
she ever had seen in her previous experiences. She also remarked, however, that "we
have more resources right at hand in the center and the community hospital than
I've ever had, too."[33]

The conditions that the nurses found in rural Bolivar County shocked them. As
the center developed, an increasing number of nurses and nurses' aides were trained
from the local population, but initially most of the nurses were white and came
from outside the South. As was the case with the center's physicians, nurses from
outside the rural South were horrified by the poverty they witnessed as they traveled
throughout the Delta. The typical home, as one nurse remembered, was "a house
made of boards, unpainted, without foundation and separate piles of rock support-
ing its four corners, surrounded on rainy days by ankle-deep mud, in dry weather by
dust. . . . The walls were papered in brown wrapping paper. . . . There was no water,
no telephone, no indoor toilet, and only the small wood-burning stove for heat. . . .
Dr. King's photograph and the stove were the two items common in all the homes
we visited."[34] Another nurse recalled entering a home in the winter to find that "the
14 people in that family all congregate in one room around a small, wood-burning
stove. . . . The floor was slick with ice where water had been tracked in and then
froze. The children were all barefoot," and "there were holes in the walls so big that
the cats came and went when they pleased."[35]

Geiger remarked that the nurses were vital to the operation of the health center
"for follow-up, for case finding, for cluing everyone else in on the home setting,
for compensating for shortages of doctors, for helping interrupt the idiot revolving-
door game, the old business of diagnosing, treating, and sending a patient right back
to the environment that produced his illness." The center sought to use its nurses—
and other health workers—for tasks not requiring a physician's special skills, thereby
providing high quality care while keeping cost and manpower demands low. Nurses
made sure that the patients were taking their prescribed medicines—and taking
the proper dosage on the right schedule; they checked on elderly patients who were
home alone; they evaluated patients and alerted physicians when someone needed to
come back to the center or be admitted for hospitalization; they reported the needs

[33] Kelly, "Health Care in the Mississippi Delta," 759–60, 762.
[34] Ibid., 760–61.
[35] Simpson, *Sister Stella's Babies*, 20.

of the rural community back to those at the center in Mound Bayou. The nurses were, in many ways, the eyes and the ears of the center out in the most rural sections of the county, and, for many of the patients, they were the face of the Tufts–Delta Health Center. "They ... would be out all day with a bag lunch, making house calls and showing new mothers how to care for their newborns," recalled one of the center's physicians, and then "they'd come back to the center and tell us where home repairs, window screens, wells, and privies were needed."[36]

Sometimes even quite serious illness was managed in a plantation shack, with the help of a home-care package designed jointly by Environmental Services Director Andy James and the center's clinicians and nurses. It consisted of a pick-up truck that delivered a hospital bed, linens, a chemical commode, and intravenous poles and tubing, for the health center nurse assigned to the case. One patient who received the home-care package was a comatose child with equine encephalitis, whose acute care, including tube feeding and range of motion exercises, was managed jointly by the mother and the nurse. The home care continued through the child's early stages of recovery, with provision of a wheelchair, and resulted in a complete return to normal function. Another recipient of the home-care package was a woman in the terminal stage of liver cancer, who lived in a plantation shack.[37]

Because of the high black infant mortality rate in Bolivar County, a major priority for the nurses both at the center and in the field was pre- and postnatal care for mothers and infants. The black infant mortality rate was not just bad, it was actually getting worse; between 1960 and 1964, the white infant mortality rate in Bolivar County decreased by 33 percent, while the black rate increased by 25 percent. Almost all black children in Bolivar County were delivered at home, not in a hospital, and by midwives—usually "granny midwives" who had never received any formal medical training. "In the city, a child is almost always born in a hospital, so if he has an early problem, he gets early care," explained Geiger. "Here, he just sickens and dies."[38] By the late-1960s, the absence of hospital delivery, combined with poor pre- and postnatal care, had created an infant and maternal mortality crisis in Bolivar County. At the time the Tufts team arrived, encouraging hospital deliveries was not a practical solution for the county's black population. For either economic or cultural reasons, most black women preferred home confinement with a midwife to going to a hospital, so the health center's leaders sought to find other means of improving the health and welfare of the county's mothers and children.

[36] Luther Carter, "Rural Health: OEO Launches Bold Mississippi Project," *Science* Vol. 156 (June 16, 1967): 1466–68; Kelly, "Health Care in the Mississippi Delta," 763; Ward interview with Dr. Helen Barnes.
[37] Jack Geiger notes, *JGC*.
[38] Lefkowitz, *Community Health Centers*, 31; Maxwell, "The Ailing Poor."

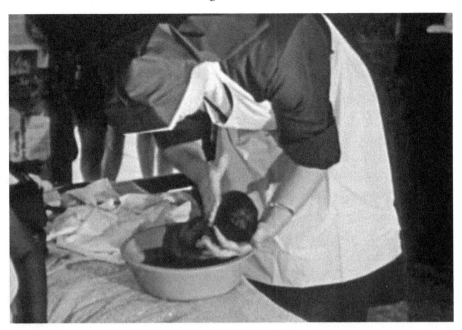

FIGURE 3.3 Sister Mary Stella Simpson tending to a newborn (Photo Credit: Victor Schoenbach).

Sister Mary Stella Simpson, a Catholic nun and registered nurse–midwife, came to Mound Bayou from Indiana at the request of the American Nurses Association when the health center was still housed in the church parsonage. In conjunction with the center, she set up a small prenatal clinic in an old storefront and began to see expectant mothers, both at the Tufts–Delta Health Center and in their homes. The days were often long—"Saw 66 patients in clinic today. Where, oh where, do they come from?" she wrote in a letter back to her order. But she persisted, traveling throughout the county, visiting expectant mothers and newborns. Working with the center's other nurse–midwife, Aase Johansen, "that nurse with the Catholic dress," as people in the county referred to Sr. Stella, delivered dozens of babies and educated mothers on their care throughout the county. If necessary, she had mothers or children admitted to the Mound Bayou Community Hospital for observation or delivery. She conducted parenting classes on breastfeeding and nutrition at the center, and also helped provide care and treatment for the infants, for things like ear infections and rashes, when they went home. Much of the focus of the center's maternal and child programs was on education and preventative care. "It's cheaper," Geiger said, "for health workers to teach mothers how to avoid contamination of water and food supplies than it is for a doctor to stay up all night giving intravenous fluids to a moribund infant."[39]

---

[39] Simpson, *Sister Stella's Babies*; Carter, "Rural Health: OEO Launches Bold Mississippi Project," 1468.

In 1968, the center hired Helen Barnes, an obstetrician–gynecologist and native Mississippian, to oversee the center's maternal and child health practice. Barnes had attended medical school at Howard University and then, like Bob Smith and Aaron Shirley, returned to Mississippi to pay off her state scholarship, setting up a practice in Greenwood. Declaring that she was "not gonna put up with this" following the murder of her friend Medgar Evers in 1963, she left Mississippi for obstetrics–gynecology training at Kings County Hospital in Brooklyn, New York. While she was finishing her residency, Geiger tried to persuade her to come back to Mississippi to establish the maternal and child program at the Tufts–Delta Health Center. She responded by telling him, "You have lost your Goddamned mind!" But the conversation did not end; "Jack can't be turned off easily," Barnes remembered. Eventually she agreed to visit the center. "When I visited the center site, it was still a hole in the ground," she recalled. "I [told Jack] I'd come back when the hole was filled. . . . When you have the clinic up and working, and it has toilets and lights in it, and all the things that I am accustomed to working with up here in New York." He held her to her word. When the permanent structure opened, Geiger again offered her a position, which she then accepted. When she arrived, she demanded some upgrades of the facilities. "For deliveries, we needed hospital space and standards," she recalled. "We took over an abandoned emergency room at the hospital, cleaned, stripped and painted the walls, scrubbed the floors, and installed screens."[40]

These maternal and infant health programs were sometimes met with resistance, however. John Hatch spent a great deal of time working with leaders in communities throughout north Bolivar County to encourage participation in the prenatal and well-baby programs offered by the health center. Initially, he found that there was little interest in such programs from mothers who did not see the need for prenatal care, and outright hostility from some of the granny midwives in the county, who saw the center as both a competitor and dismissive of their service and knowledge. In order to try to assuage the hostility and garner support for the health center's programs, Hatch met with some of the granny midwives. He described meeting with one 70-year-old midwife from Alligator, whom he recalled as having "strong anti-center views." She told him that she had delivered two out of every three black people under 40 years of age living in the community, and that "taking care of sick babies . . . required a loving heart as well as an understanding of their bodies." He eventually convinced her to sit down and talk about the infant mortality problem in the area and described to her what was being done at the center. He told her

[40] Barnes interview with Ward; Lefkowitz, *Community Health Centers*, 38.

that there were two nurse–midwives working at the health center, and asked for her advice on what types of programs she thought the center should undertake to improve the health of mothers and babies. Taken aback, she smiled and said, "So you finally found out we have some sense after all." Hatch assured her that he valued her input, and encouraged her to join the Alligator Health Association. She did, became co-chairman of its mother and child committee, and eventually her home was placed on the center's list of approved places to shelter children during family crises.[41]

In order get more mothers, and mothers-to-be, to take part in the center's pre-natal programs, and to encourage local leadership on health issues, meetings were organized throughout the county by the local health associations. Hatch found that attendance at these meetings increased when they were led by community members instead of center staff, and when topics were not just focused on health issues, but oriented toward other interests of mothers, such as dressmaking, grooming, or food preparation. Hatch also found other ways to put the health center's message into the association meetings, without driving people away. For example, the staff nutrition-ist would prepare a special dish for the social hour, which gave her an opportunity to explain new and healthy ways to prepare foods, without subjecting people to a lecture on nutrition. Similarly, sessions focusing on "How to help your child suc-ceed," eventually led to discussions of health issues, such as vaccinations, the impor-tance of which members of the center's staff had been having difficulty impressing on many mothers.[42]

The combination of improved medical intervention from the center's specialists, combined with the community outreach that brought both the traditional birth at-tendants and the mothers on board with the center's nutrition and pre- and postna-tal programs were a spectacular success, reducing the black infant mortality rate by 50 percent in north Bolivar County during the center's first two years. The Tufts–Delta Health Center's program made such great strides that the *American Journal of Nursing* reported that, "From an almost universal lack of any prenatal care three years ago, the trend now is to attendance at the center's ante-natal clinic, often before the fifth month of pregnancy, delivery at the community hospital, postpartum follow-up, and protection of infants from birth on. 'Quite a change' [Mrs. Walker] says, 'from the days when Sr. Mary Stella and Aase Johansson [*sic.*] saw many moth-ers for the first time when they were ready to deliver—or had delivered—and from

---

[41] North Bolivar County farm cooperative self-help nutritional program. Grant proposal written by John Hatch, 1972, *JHC*.
[42] Ibid.

the time when little children never saw a doctor or nurse until they were so ill with diarrhea or pneumonia that it was touch and go to save them.' "[43]

In addition to maternal and infant health, family planning was another major initiative of the health center, albeit one fraught with a host of delicate issues. By the late-1960s, sterilization and birth control had become very controversial subjects among African Americans, especially in Mississippi, which had a sordid history of involuntary sterilization of black women by white physicians. Hatch recounted stories of local women who were required by county officials to have what was termed "a little operation" after an out-of-wedlock pregnancy if they wanted to remain on the welfare rolls. The "Mississippi appendectomy," a hysterectomy administered to black women who came in for other surgery, was conducted on thousands of black women in the Jim Crow South, and came to national attention when the civil rights icon Fannie Lou Hamer, from neighboring Sunflower County, testified about her experience with forced sterilization. Even voluntary birth control was a sensitive issue at the time, because numerous black leaders viewed cheap—or free—birth control administered to black women by the government as a means of racial genocide; indeed, in 1962, the National Urban League actually rescinded its support for birth control, as did a number of NAACP chapters.[44]

Given the sensitive culture surrounding birth control in Mississippi, a family-planning program for poor black women in the Delta—one administered by white physicians from the North, no less—was an especially delicate proposition. The need, however, was undeniable: Large families had been a necessity during the sharecropping era, when many hands were viewed as an economic asset, but as that economy dissolved large families became a financial liability and a danger to the health of mothers. (Both the region's poverty and high infant and maternal mortality rates bore these facts out starkly.) So, while appreciating the potential pitfalls, Christian Hansen decided to establish a family-planning program. He was assisted at the clinic's family planning service by two black staff physicians, because, as Hansen put it, "there were political sensitivities back then to having a white man help black women have fewer children." Nonetheless, Hansen observed that his patients "were glad to have the power to control their fertility."[45]

Hansen, a pediatrician, traveled to New York to learn how to insert intrauterine devices and prescribe the birth control pill. Despite some opposition, especially from older women in the community who believed that large families were ordained by God, during the program's first year, Hansen treated 154 women,

---

[43] Kelly, "Health Care in the Mississippi Delta," 762.

[44] Harriet A. Washington, *Medical Apartheid* (New York: Doubleday, 2006), 189–90, 198, 202; John Hatch narrative, *JHC*.

[45] Hansen, *In the Name of the Children*, 71.

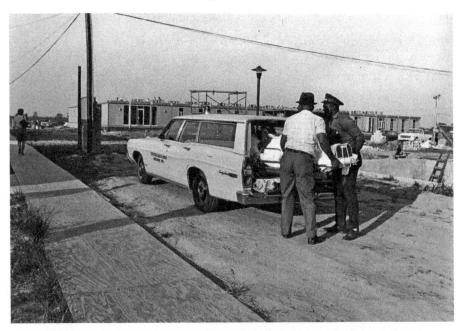

FIGURE 3.4 Transporting a patient to the Tufts–Delta Health Center (Photo courtesy of Dan Bernstein, Southern Historical Collection, University of North Carolina at Chapel Hill).

ranging in age from fourteen to forty-two, who had had an average of 5.5 pregnancies before birth control was administered. Two-thirds of the women were enrolled in the program at the time of their postpartum exams at the health center, while the remaining women signed on after bringing their children to the pediatrician for care. Hansen found that some of them had previously sought out birth control, and had even used the pill for a short period of time, but were either unable to afford it or had been unable to obtain it from a local physician, leading Hansen to comment that, "These experiences point out the importance of a comprehensive health program which removes cost as a barrier to obtaining healthcare." When Dr. Helen Barnes joined the center's staff in 1968, Hansen turned the program over to her.[46]

By early 1969, less than two years after the Tufts–Delta Health Center began operating, *LIFE* magazine reported that the center had treated more than 8,000 patients in northern Bolivar County, and the nursing staff alone had made more than 10,000 home visits. By then the health center had a staff of ten physicians, ten nurses, two trained midwives, and a professional staff that included social workers, clinical technicians, a nutritionist, and a pharmacist; twenty-nine members of the professional staff were black. The center also employed a clinical psychologist, Dr. Florence

---

[46] Hansen, "The Pediatrician and Family Planning in a Very Poor Community," 320–22.

Halpern, who provided mental health services and did social work. Halpern found a significant amount of depression among those served by the center, particularly women. "It may be because you can't raise five dollars for a new dress, because you can't pick cotton anymore, or it might be a minor physical ailment that is gone untreated," Halpern told *The Wall Street Journal* in 1969. "Or because the house is empty, with the man and grown children moved north." She tried to help women cope with depression by "organizing group sessions for the women so they can sew or knit themselves a dress and get together with other women in the same boat." Her successes at the center, especially in working with women and youths, soon attracted the attention of local white mayors and police chiefs throughout Bolivar County, who regularly brought her in as a consultant on issues involving African Americans in their towns. Halpern often negotiated arrangements under which the police referred adolescents in trouble to her rather than involve them in juvenile justice detention systems.[47]

Although the Tufts–Delta Health Center grew out of the civil rights movement and was located in an all-black town, its founders always hoped that it would serve all the poor in north Bolivar County, no matter what their race. Despite this hope, the center attracted few white patients to its doors, even though there was a significant impoverished white population in the area in desperate need of its services. The center's inability to attract white patients was, of course, a legacy of segregation: No white person—no matter how poor—was likely to associate themselves with any black institutions, lest they be ostracized by the white community. Tied to this white aversion to the center was the belief held by most Mississippi whites that virtually all War on Poverty programs were nothing more than "nigger programs" designed to promote black civil rights.

Ultimately, due to both outreach and need, some whites did begin to use the center's services, including Pearlie Johnson, a widow with two daughters who lived on $1,500 a year. She had developed cataracts, but did not even seek out medical help because, in her words, "Town doctors don't take up with us poor folks." Soon after the health center opened, she went for help, despite admonitions from friends about "takin' up with black folks"; she even had to quit her church because other members harassed her about going to Mound Bayou. The health center paid for her treatment by an eye doctor in Greenville, and Willie Dixon, a social worker at the center—who was black—visited the Johnson home every week.[48]

---

[47] Hall, "A Stir of Hope in Mound Bayou," 73; Maxwell, "The Ailing Poor"; Interview with H. Jack Geiger by Kornstad and Boothby.

[48] Joseph J. Huttie Jr., "New Federalism and the Death of a Dream in Mound Bayou, Mississippi," *New South* 28:4 (Fall 1973): 20–29.

Another area where the center struggled, despite its early successes, was in enticing medical professionals to come, and stay, in Mound Bayou. The isolation and poverty of the region, along with Mississippi's reputation for intolerance and violence, made the Tufts–Delta Health Center a tough sell for Geiger when trying to attract doctors and other professionals. Although the federally funded center could offer a fair wage for its professional staff, the pay was still below what most would make on the open market, and the lack of amenities in and around Mound Bayou was a very difficult pill for most recruits—especially those with young families, many of whom were concerned with employment opportunities for spouses and schools for their children.

Housing was an especially acute problem for the center's staff. Initial plans to build staff housing near the center never materialized. Some staff bought or rented homes in nearby Cleveland, while most, including Jack Geiger, lived in trailers on empty lots in and around Mound Bayou. Christian Hansen paid $5,000 for a supposedly new trailer to house his family, only to arrive and find it badly dented and situated on a rented yard with broken glass, abandoned cars, and old tires. Still, Hansen conceded, "We were lucky to have indoor plumbing. We also had a washer/dryer, and, most importantly, air conditioning."[49]

The social and professional isolation of Mound Bayou was a constant challenge for the health center's staff and their families. Leon Kruger's wife taught at the local Mound Bayou high school for several years, and some other wives of the professional staff also worked or volunteered at local schools, but the social and cultural gap was difficult for many of them to overcome. Hansen recalled that soon after arriving in town, "We began to learn about the depth and complexity of race relations in Mound Bayou. . . . There was an enormous social gulf between the black people and white professionals from out-of-state. The only unforced socializing was among the mixed staff at the Health Center. John Hatch . . . was the main catalyst. . . . His children and ours played together after getting over their initial shyness." Even Hatch, who was black and a native Southerner, was still seen as an outsider by locals because of his education and time spent in the North. Sometimes the cultural divide made for humorous exchanges between the staff and the locals; when Geiger was unable to distinguish between a soybean field and

---

[49] H. J. Geiger, "A Health Center for Social Change: People and Poverty in Rural Mississippi," Supplementary Text published by *Network for Continuing Medical Education*, New York, June 1971, p. 24; Hansen, *In the Name of the Children*, 56–58.

Leon Kruger's daughter, Jo Ivester, wrote a memoir *The Outskirts of Hope*, based on her memories and her mother's journal from their family's time in Mound Bayou. It provides a number of interesting insights into the difficulties that the families faced.

a cotton field, the locals were shocked. "But he's a doctor!" they said. "Where'd he go to school?"[50]

Geiger and his team were able to overcome these obstacles and successfully recruit a highly motivated, top-notch staff to come to the Delta. Some, like Chris Hansen and Mary Clifford, a cardiologist from Michigan, were white Northerners who came to the center because of their dedication to civil rights and social justice, while others, like Helen Barnes and Harvey Sanders, a surgeon, were native black Mississippians who saw in the Tufts–Delta Health Center a way to give back to the most poverty-stricken residents of their home state. John Hatch recalled that recruiting black professionals was a great challenge—"I don't think we were ever able to get a northern black person to come for a professional job," he remarked—but the center did attract some African Americans like himself and Helen Barnes who had migrated north and decided to return south for the purpose of working at the health center. As Barnes later remarked, "The civil rights movement . . . gave them hope to believe that the South could become a viable place to practice." Hatch later stated that, "For me, it was the first time I could see the possibility of some credible change happening through efforts that I might carry out, and carry out in dignity."[51]

Even the most dedicated activists, however, lasted at most a few years at the center. Helen Barnes stayed in Mound Bayou for two years before moving to the University of Mississippi Medical Center in Jackson; she said that the isolation of Mound Bayou got to her. Christian Hansen later wrote that, "After a year of working in this cutting-edge project fighting poverty, a despondency took hold of me. . . . I became irritable with Alix [his wife] and bothered by our children and their friends. At work, I was less willing to extend myself to provide night coverage. One night I . . . told Alix, 'I can't function anymore.'" A psychiatrist Geiger sent from Tufts to speak to Hansen advised him to return home. Hansen's wife and children returned to Pennsylvania while he finished the last months of his term at the center. He left Mound Bayou in 1969 and went on to direct an inner city health center in Trenton, New Jersey.[52]

Recruiting replacement staff was "a constant, unending task," remembered Geiger. He took out ads in journals and newspapers, and traveled the country telling people about the Mississippi project, all the while trying to entice talented applicants to come to the Mississippi Delta. When Leon Kruger, the health center's first clinical director, departed with his family, Geiger secured as his replacement

---

[50] Hansen, *In the Name of the Children*, 58–60: Sobelson, "Participation, Power, and Place," 65–66.

[51] Sobelson, "Participation, Power, and Place," 66–67; Ward interview with John Hatch and Jack Geiger.

[52] Lefkowiz, *Community Health Centers*, 38; Hansen, *In the Name of the Children*, 76.

Dr. David Weeks, who had for several years directed a large oil company hospital in Saudi Arabia. Weeks had decided to return to the United States to rejoin mainstream medicine and provide a good education for his young children. Geiger convinced him that what was happening in Bolivar County was the cutting-edge of medical progress in the United States and recruited him as clinical director, a post he occupied for many years.

Similarly, when John Hatch and his family left for Chapel Hill, North Carolina, in 1971 so he could pursue his doctorate in public health, Hatch successfully recruited Ted Parrish, an experienced social worker and community organizer in North Carolina, to replace him as head of the Community Health Action staff. A succession of black administrators for the health center, including Paul Reese from Baltimore and C. E. Prothro from Atlanta, occupied important management positions throughout the late 1960s and early 1970s.[53]

In a system somewhat similar to the partnership between Meharry and the Taborian Hospital/Mound Bayou Community Hospital, Tufts Medical School also provided some staffing for the health center by allowing its senior year students and faculty to travel to Mississippi to work at the center as part of the school's curriculum. Their work focused on public health issues and the connections between social conditions and ill health. Each Tufts student who traveled to Mound Bayou was assigned to a family health care group—an interdisciplinary team consisting of a pediatrician, an internist, a social worker, and a community health nurse—as was done at Columbia Point in Boston. Although this program provided both valuable training for Tufts medical students and helped alleviate the staffing demands at the health center, it came under criticism from some local black leaders (many of whom were already opposed to the center) who argued that this program showed what they had always suspected—that the health center was little more than a training facility for Tufts medical students who were using Mound Bayou as a laboratory for Third World medical instruction.[54]

Because of the difficulties in both recruiting and retaining professional staff, it was not until the center's 1970–1971 grant year that it could report that "for the first time in its history, [the center is operating] with a full complement of young, well-trained generalists; internists; pediatricians; obstetrician–gynecologists; and a surgeon." The center's nursing department, however, was still not quite at full strength that year.[55] Despite the staffing difficulties, by this time the health center had, indeed, begun to fulfill much of the promise that Geiger and others had for it

[53] Jack Geiger notes, *JGC.*
[54] Carter, "Rural Health: OEO Launches Bold Mississippi Project," 1468.
[55] Geiger, "A Health Center for Social Change," 24.

when they envisioned it five years earlier. Health care delivery throughout northern Bolivar County had awakened the staff to the greater needs of the community—food, housing, clothing, employment, and empowerment; needs that the Tufts–Delta Health Center sought to cater to as well.

By 1970, the paraprofessional staff was overwhelmingly recruited and trained from members of the local community, providing educational and economic opportunities that had not existed before and in many ways fulfilled the OEO's mandate of "maximum feasible participation by the poor" in ways that the federal government had never envisioned. In addition to positions in health care delivery, as it expanded its scope of operations, the health center created employment opportunities for many locals outside of traditional health care. Through environmental services, a food co-op, child-care centers, a bookstore, and other services created throughout northern Bolivar County, the Tufts–Delta Health Center was a catalyst for more than just improved health care in the region; it brought hope and empowerment for a population that had been sadly lacking in both before the center arrived.

A community's health status is a function of its environmental health, its economic
health, its mental health, and educational health, and then physical health. Unless
you had those things in balance, it's hard to get a healthy community.
DR. ANDREW JAMES[1]

Penicillin may be indicated to cure pneumonia, but it alone will not stop the roof from leaking
DR. ROY BROWN[2]

4

Environmental Factors

FROM THE INCEPTION of the Tufts–Delta Health Center, Jack Geiger expressed
an expansive vision of health care that went far beyond treatment of the sick and
basic preventative care. Instead, he saw the health center to be "designed as a base for
multiple points of entry into the problems of health and poverty," including water,
sanitation facilities, and protection from the environment in housing fit for human
habitation.[3]

In his time in Mississippi, Geiger saw that the conditions that many impoverished
people lived in dramatically impacted their health, recalling that "black people . . .
lived in crumbling, patchwork shacks with leaking roofs, rotting floors, buckling
walls, gaping windows, newspaper for insulation and crude stoves for heating and
cooking—when there was firewood. Many drank contaminated water from drainage ditches and used dilapidated surface privies. . . . Infants, under such circumstances, often ingested their own excrement; children lacked the shoes to walk to
school, the clothes to wear, or . . . the food to sustain learning."

These living conditions made the medical care administered at the health center
useless unless the surrounding environmental conditions also were improved.
Geiger therefore became convinced that one of the priorities of the health center

---

[1] Andrew James interview with Tom Ward.
[2] Brown, "Delivery of Pediatric Health Services in A Rural Health Center."
[3] Geiger, "A Health Center for Social Change: People and Poverty in Rural Mississippi."

was to develop an environmental division to go out into the towns, hamlets, and plantation shacks of Bolivar County to improve basic living conditions. As Geiger wrote in 1971, "Most of the critical health problems suffered by this population (infant and maternal mortality, malnutrition, infectious disease, tuberculosis) have long since been solved in affluent America. Their persistence in poverty areas suggests that conventional and narrowly restrictive 'medical' techniques and programs are an insufficient answer."[4]

When the Tufts–Delta Health Center sought to hire a full-time sanitarian, Geiger was committed to recruiting an African American for the position. In order to do so, John Hatch, then the program director of the health center, called the Association of Professional Sanitarians to ask after black members, and found that there were very few. Hatch eventually contacted Andrew James, a Birmingham, Alabama, native who had received his Master's in Environmental Engineering from the University of Cincinnati in 1967 and was currently working in the health department in Dayton, Ohio. James visited the center and decided to take the position. "I wanted to get to where the need was . . . and to get a hand on where the problem was, in the South," he later recalled. "As a black man I was paying some dues."[5] James, a tall, soft-spoken, elegant man—whose nickname the "Rat Man" could only have been derived from the trappings of his work—proved to be everything that Geiger and Hatch were looking for in someone to direct the center's environmental health program. During his tenure at the Tufts–Delta Health Center, first as director of the environmental health division, and later as the center's director, James was not only able to work with the local black communities in dramatically improving their health conditions and bringing about sanitary reforms for the people of Bolivar County, he was also extremely effective—in a way that many of the other leaders of the health center were not—in working with local white leaders, most of whom were openly hostile to the Tufts–Delta Health Center and its programs.

Access to clean water was one of the most pressing issues confronting black communities when James arrived in Mound Bayou, and it had a direct impact on health. "They were losing babies here because of infectious diarrhea and bad water," he recalled. At that time, only 29 percent of the black population in Bolivar County had piped water. Instead, they relied on pumps, hydrants, or hauled water. James discovered that many of the black residents of the county used discarded 55-gallon drums, most of which had been used to transport chemicals, including DDT and other pesticides used on the plantations, to store water that they hauled from

[4] Geiger, "A Health Center for Social Change: People and Poverty in Rural Mississippi."
[5] Interview with Andy James, Delta Health Center Tapes, (Disk 1, Reel 5–5).

municipal water supplies miles away. Others gathered water from irrigation ditches. Even homes that did have pumps, James found, did not get clean water because the wells did not go deep enough. "One of the problems has been that the residents of our target population will get water from about 12 feet," he later recalled. "You can get water from about 12 feet, especially if you're close to the river . . . but this type of water is simply not fit to drink . . . [and those] wells dry up when the river flow begins to fall."[6]

One of the major obstacles that James and his team initially ran into was simply convincing local people that their water was the source of many of their health problems. "Clear water is good water," was what people believed, no matter where the water came from. John Hatch credited an educational program run by a local man employed by the health center for changing minds and gaining support for the environmental health programs. Murray Nelson was "not a literate person," according to Hatch, but he was "mechanically gifted in the assembly and maintenance of complex machines," and "he gave the most effective presentations on environmental health I've ever witnessed." Traveling throughout the county with the environmental health team, Hatch recalled that "Murray set up displays and presented slide presentations of local pests and parasites invisible to the human eye. He would present a glass of clear water and asked the audience if they saw any reason not to drink it. . . . He would then say that the particular glass of water was full of disease . . . and people would laugh." Nelson then prepared a slide from the water sample and invited his audience—most of whom had never looked through a microscope before—to come and take a look. Most gasped when they saw all the living organisms crawling around in their water. "Their wonder provided teachable moments," recalled Hatch, and was an essential part of convincing people to allow the environmental health team to come in and work with them.[7]

"Ironically," Andrew James reported, "Bolivar County has an abundance of ground water. Unfortunately, most rural poor cannot afford pumping equipment if a well exceeding 35 feet must be developed." To alleviate this problem, James and his team developed a two-man pump-diver system to provide potable water for area residents. "The Mississippi River is about 20 miles from here," noted James, "and I recognized that would be enough hydrostatic pressure to push that water through to this area." So his team "took a ¾ inch pipe and filled it with concrete," then they took a sawed-off telephone pole, put two handles on the side of it, and "my workers would stand on each side and drive pipe in the ground." Eventually, "pure water came out. . . .

---

[6] Andy James interview with Tom Ward, June 8, 2013; "Bolivar County Census Highlights (prepared for Tufts), 1968," Collection 4613, Series 1, Subseries 1, Box 3, Folder 23, *DHC*; Interview with Andy James, Delta Health Center Tapes.

[7] John Hatch narrative, *JHC.*

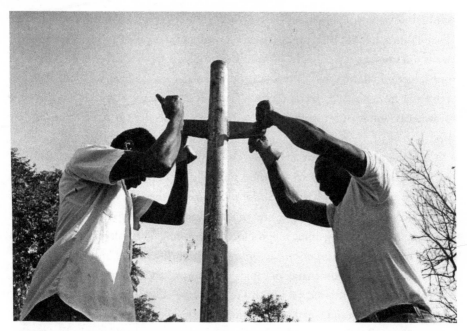

FIGURE 4.1 Drilling for water (Photo courtesy of Dan Bernstein, Southern Historical Collection, University of North Carolina at Chapel Hill).

So we just got the old-fashioned pump . . . and then people could pump water." In search of a better, more sustainable solution to the water problem, James secured funding for a proper well-digging machine, and, as Geiger recalled, "all over Bolivar County you would see these orange-handed pumps that we had installed as a simple protected well for water."[8]

In addition to the lack of clean drinking water, sewage disposal was a major health issue for black residents of the region. When the health center opened, it was estimated that 90 percent of African Americans living in north Bolivar County had no flush toilet; the most common method of rural home sewage disposal was the "sunshine privy"—basically an outhouse, minus a pit or rear wall. Small cesspools with no secondary treatment—little more than holes in the ground—served as the next most common system of home sewage disposal. "It was just a bad scene—to a person, to a sanitarian, to an environmental engineer—to see something like this," James recalled. The negative health effects of such improper facilities were obvious, and providing both immediate and long-term solutions for the proper disposal of human waste became a priority for James. Faced with both the poor existing

---

[8] Dr. Andy James, "The Organization of an Environmental Health Unit in a Comprehensive Health Services Center," presented at OEO Training Conference, 1970. Collection 4613. Box 20, Folder 146, *DHC*; Andy James interview with Tom Ward; Interview with H. Jack Geiger by Robert Korstad and Neil Boothby.

conditions and the extreme poverty of the area, James admitted that he "had to shift my values down," and initially focused on immediate solutions to try and improve environmental health conditions in the area.[9]

As they had with the pipe-driving team, James and his men began by using relatively primitive methods to improve sewage conditions, beginning by simply tearing down old, dilapidated privies and building sanitary ones in their place. "We're doing a great deal of basic sanitation here, we can't get sophisticated at all," he told one interviewer. "I would say it's probably similar to some underdeveloped countries, in terms of keeping the waste, a person's waste, from being ingested again." One of the problems that James found in building new privies was that even though most of his "clients" lived on large plantations, there was often very little space allocated by the landowners for the tenants, so he often had to build the new privies closer to the tenant's home than he thought safe. "You have a problem because the plantation, most of its land is to grow something, so you can get a profit on it, and so you could usually find only about 400 square foot to furnish that whole family for all of its needs in terms of getting rid of its waste, getting its water, recreation, housing space, and getting rid of its solid waste in terms of garbage," recalled James.[10]

Building new privies for people living in mid-twentieth century America, however, was not an acceptable solution for either Andy James or Jack Geiger. The lack of sewers in black communities, especially in Delta cities and towns, forced James and the Tufts–Delta Health Center into both legal and political fights to improve and modernize sewage systems for black Mississippians. This was, essentially, an extension of the civil rights movement, but for clean water and sanitary communities instead of access to public facilities and the ballot. As James surveyed the region, he found that "the existence of sewered white areas and non-sewered black areas . . . is widespread. Essentially, the black man is taxed to support an important health service for whites and he is denied it."

In Pace, a town in the health center's target area of northern Bolivar County, "the entire town is serviced by a water system under pressure. The White community is sewered by discharging untreated septic tank effluents, collected in an underground sewage system, into one of the two streams running through the town. The Black community relies on outdoor pit privies or, for those with indoor toilets, on discharging septic tank effluents into street quarters."[11] At this time the United States had twice

---

[9] Dr. Andy James, "The Organization of an Environmental Health Unit in a Comprehensive Health Services Center"; Interview with Andy James, Delta Health Center Tapes.

[10] Interview with Andy James, Delta Health Center Tapes.

[11] James, "The Organization of an Environmental Health Unit. . ."; Howard, S. J., "Report of a Work Project in the Environmental Services Division of Tufts–Delta Health Center, Mound Bayou, Mississippi."

landed men on the moon, and brought them home safely, yet human waste was still running in the streets of black sections of Mississippi towns.

In response to these inequities, representatives from the Tufts–Delta Health Center partnered with local residents on lawsuits to bring sewer services to their communities. The center had its own legal department and worked with lawyers from the American Civil Liberties Union (ACLU), the National Association for the Advancement of Colored People (NAACP), and Tufts University in bringing lawsuits. In a landmark case, *Hawkins v. Shaw [Miss.]* (1971), a federal court ruled that southern cities must equalize funding for public services—such as paved roads, fire hydrants, sidewalks, streetlights, and water and sewer systems—in black and white neighborhoods. The case established a precedent for the creation of equal municipal facilities across the South.[12]

Representatives of the health center and the health council met repeatedly with the lead attorney in the case, the NAACP's Mel Leventhal, who encouraged them to bring similar suits in their own communities as *Shaw* slowly made its way through the justice system. In Rosedale, black residents were inspired to take to the streets to boycott downtown businesses to force the city to provide sewerage for the black section of town. In 1965 Rosedale had the highest infant mortality rate in northern Bolivar County, and a 1970 study done by John Hatch found that nearly 90 percent of the black children in Rosedale and its environs had worms, and a third showed signs of malnutrition. "Rosedale's population had a black majority," recalls Geiger, "but of course the town government was lily-white. The white part of town was pretty; the black part had dirt roads, no sidewalks, no sewer system. Whenever it rained heavily, Rosedale's streets were literally awash with feces."[13]

In 1970 the Rosedale Health Association, working in cooperation with the Tufts–Delta Health Center, sponsored efforts to alert citizens to the health hazards connected with the raw sewage that ran through black Rosedale. The outreach encompassed efforts to mobilize and politicize citizens and to quantify scientifically the disease and sickness that already had been wrought by the sewage problem. Environmental health staff from the health center came to Rosedale to collect water and soil samples for testing, then prepared cultures showing contaminated water

[12] Memo of Meeting with Attorney Mel Leventhal, March 24, 1971, Box 20, Folder 147, *DHC*; Roy Reed, "Equal Service Edict Irks Town," *New York Times*, March 2, 1971; Andy James interview with Tom Ward.

[13] John Hatch and Anita P Holmes, "Rural and Small Town African-American Populations and Human Rights in Postindustrial Society," in Marion Gray Secundy, Ed., *Bioethics Research Concerns and Directions for African-Americans* (Tuskegee University, 2000): pp. 68–80; H. Jack Geiger, "Voting is Good For Your Health!" Guest blog, Campaign for America's Health Centers, March 12, 2102 http://blog.saveourchcs.org/2012/03/29/voting-is-good-for-your-health/; John Hatch narrative, *JHC*.

and soil. Medical personnel provided educational programs to explain the health effects of drinking contaminated water, and examined over 200 people for health problems.[14] Jack Cartwright was a community development worker with the Tufts–Delta Health Center at the time of the Rosedale outreach; he recalled that "the community found expression through the Health Association." In addition to the sewage problem, the black community of Rosedale, now energized for change, drew up a list of concerns that they presented to the town officials, merchants, and the broader white community. They called for an ample supply of chlorinated water in the black community; the need to enact and enforce a housing code; road repair and a better lighting systems in the poorer neighborhoods; improved recreational facilities; the need for the town's merchants to hire more black employees, and to change their attitudes and practices toward their black customers; and, finally, the need to improve relationships between the police and the black community, including the hiring of a proportional representation of black officers. Cartwright reported that although a few meetings were held with city leaders, the merchants and town officials "did not show a willingness to recognize the problems" of the black community. As a result, the Rosedale Health Association, along with church and club leaders, called for a boycott of downtown businesses in order to get the city fathers to recognize the legitimacy of their grievances.[15] Environmental health had become a new face of the civil rights movement, at least in this part of Mississippi.

The involvement of members of the Tufts–Delta Health Center in economic protests was a dicey proposition. As a federally funded, OEO program, the center was banned from participating in political activities, including boycotts. Its workers could, of course, engage in political activities on their own time, but not during working hours, and they could not use government cars for any type of political activity. This prohibition on political action had always been a difficult pill for Geiger to swallow, because he saw political power as coming with a responsibility to provide for good health. Since the inception of the health center, Geiger had maintained that to succeed it had to do more than merely treat people's physical ailments; the center had to dramatically alter the concept of what health care entailed, as well as empower local people to take an active role in the improvement of their communities. Having been deeply involved in civil rights activities before joining the health center, Geiger believed in the importance of political action to bring about change. Barbara Brooks, a native of Bolivar County and an employee at the health center, recalled that the center's staff encouraged members of the local population to become active in bringing

---

[14] Memo—"August Outreach in Rosedale," Box 60, Folder 432a, *DHC*.
[15] Jack Cartwright, "Health Association Progress Reports, 1971," Box 38, Folder 285, *DHC*.

about change in their communities. The contact, or satellite, centers established by the health associations became hubs of political activity, where people learned how to demand change from their political officials. "[They were] where people would go and have meetings and talk about the problems that was existing in their town," Brooks recalled.[16]

Although health center employees encouraged local residents to become involved in local affairs, including registering to vote, the Tufts–Delta Health Center risked losing its federal funding if it became overtly embroiled in political movements. This fact was not lost on opponents of the health center, and these parties sought to use any health center involvement in the Rosedale boycott as a means to have the Tufts–Delta Health Center stripped of its federal appropriations. The Mississippi State Sovereignty Commission, which regularly monitored members of the center's staff because of their past civil rights activities, assigned one of its spies, James M. Mohead, to observe the activities in Rosedale. Mohead reported that "[Rosedale] Mayor Lawler is of the opinion that the boycott is being conducted under the direction of Tufts Medical Center," given that "Johnny L. Todd . . . an employee of Tufts, is openly directing the pickets. Mayor Lawler advised that he believes pickets are being paid with Tufts funds." The report went on further to allege that a Sovereignty Commission source "advised that pickets are being paid $4 to $5 per day for carrying picket signs. They are paid by Jack Cartwright [of the Tufts–Delta Health Center], but the money source is not known. . . . Source advised that a car pool has been organized to transport negroes to surrounding towns in order to purchase groceries. Persons who provide cars for this pool are reportedly being paid $3 to $5 per trip." In later reports, the agent was frustrated by his inability to link any direct health center involvement to the boycott, expressing frustration that there was a "gross misuse" of forty U.S. government cars by Tufts employees, but "since the duty of these drivers is to travel throughout the country transporting patients to and from the Medical Center and other negroes to the various contact points, it has been impossible to establish whether or not they are on official business."[17]

The Rosedale boycott went on for three months without resolving the main issues at hand, but it was successful in raising the consciousness of both the city's white leaders to the demands of their black citizens and of the black community itself.

---

[16] Interview with Barbara Brooks and Jack Cartwright by Martha Minette, Rosedale, Mississippi (1999), Southern Historical Collection, UNC-Chapel Hill.

[17] James M. Mohead, "Weekly Reports" [SCR ID # 99-1-0-12-1-1-1 and 99-1-0-14-1-1-1], *MSC*.

James defended both the boycott and the role of health center employees in it. In a letter to Rosedale's white leadership, he wrote:

> The center is aware of the boycott currently being waged by the black community of Rosedale. Some of the people involved in the boycott may in fact be employees of this center. Our records indicate that they do not directly participate in the boycott during their hours of work. . . . One of the premises of the Community Action Program is that poverty can be overcome as the poor gain the capability to play an effective role in the community processes that affect them. . . . [The] Tufts–Delta Health Center would in no way dictate to a community who its leaders should be. That is clearly up to the community.[18]

In May 1972, Rosedale was awarded a $148,000 grant to upgrade its water and sewage facilities, and extend full service to all parts of the town. The new water and sewage system would eventually be completed under the administration of Johnny Todd, and the first black mayor of the town, former employee of the Tufts–Delta Health Center who led the boycott.[19]

Lawsuits and protests like those in Rosedale were confrontational means of addressing the lack of sewerage in the Mississippi Delta, but Andrew James also worked with public officials on the city, county, and state level to improve health conditions through cooperation. Indeed, one of the main factors that allowed Rosedale and other Delta towns to modernize their water and sewer systems, for all citizens, was the influx of federal grant money, which James worked tirelessly to procure. "I worked with the governor of the state . . . [and] his sanitary engineers," James said in an interview. "Money was the thing," stated James, but "we would never have been able to do all those things without some people on both sides understanding that we have to work together. And now you can see the standpipes all over Bolivar County and a lot of that came through those meetings."[20]

The ability to work across racial lines was a strength of Andy James's, first as Director of Environmental Health and later as the Director of the Tufts–Delta Health Center itself, a post he assumed in November 1969. He discussed the difficulties of getting local whites on board with his program in a 1969 article, writing, "Most Southern whites are hostile to outsiders, especially black people, who they consider workers of change," but that he found that "the hostility of whites was often replaced by interest when they discover the public health was the issue rather than civil rights." One of the

---

[18] Letter from Andrew James, Health Center Director, to M. J. Dattel, Nov. 2, 1970, Series 1, Subseries 1, Box 1, Folder 3, *DHC*;

[19] "Rosedale to get $148,000, *Delta Democrat-Times*, May 28, 1972.

[20] Andy James interview with Tom Ward, June 8, 2013.

areas where James was able to work with local white authorities was in developing an effective mosquito control program. As mosquito eradication programs run by the health center began throughout north Bolivar County—through fogging, employing larvasides, and draining stagnant water sites—James found that local whites would contact him and request that he also treat their neighborhoods as well, because many of the local governments were not involved in mosquito eradication at all. "This allows us another point of entry, and it also gives us some access with the white community, because they get bitten just as surely as the black community," James reported. "That means we have to speak to the white mayors and city councilman and try to do something about problems that affect the whole community."[21]

Eradicating all types of disease-carrying vermin was a major focus of the center's environmental health program, and James initiated a number of programs to fumigate houses, clean up garbage dumps, and kill rats and snakes. Again, the lack of basic infrastructure in waste removal was an obstacle. "Existing services that you would expect in a normal community just isn't here," he reported in 1969. There was no garbage pickup in the black communities of Bolivar County, and incinerators and sanitary landfills were rare anywhere in the state. "Municipal open dumps and wayside dumping by individuals is the usual method of solid waste disposal, and the population of rats and other vermin that find food and harbor in these dumps defies imagination," James recalled.[22]

The lack of garbage pickup also increased the population of mosquitoes and flies, and the dilapidated homes were usually no barrier to keeping vermin out. Thus, as the Environmental Health Unit engaged in vector control throughout the region—fumigating for bugs and poisoning rats and other vermin—they realized that without improvements to housing, they were fighting a useless battle. The vast majority of African Americans in north Bolivar County were sharecroppers—or former sharecroppers—who lived in plantation shacks. One newspaper reporter described the conditions he found when he visited the health center in 1971:

> It's not unusual in Mississippi . . . for a family with six or nine children to live
> in a three room house with a pump in the backyard near a three-sided toilet
> that has no roof. . . . The roofs of corrugated metal or tar-paper leak, the sides
> are patched with roadside advertising signs, screens are missing from windows
> and often lack panes, and flies and mosquitoes find easy entry, as do the field
> rats that come through the holes in walls and floors.[23]

---

[21] Ward interview with James; James, "The Organization of an Environmental Health Unit. . .," 439.

[22] James, "The Organization of an Environmental Health Unit. . .," 439, 444; Interview with Andy James, Delta Health Center Tapes; Hall, "A Stir of Hope in Mound Bayou."

[23] McDaniel, "Community Health Centers More Than Clinics for the Poor."

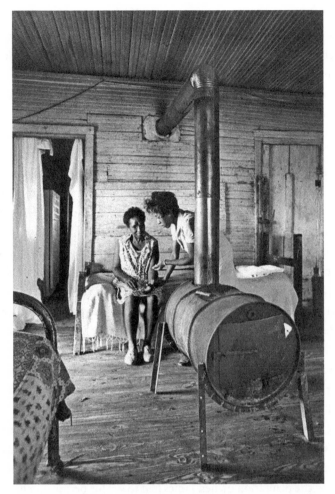

FIGURE 4.2 A nurse from the Tufts–Delta Health Center treats a patient in her home. Stoves like the one pictured, made from 55-gallon drums, provided the only heat for many sharecropper shacks in north Bolivar County and throughout the Mississippi Delta. Physicians from the health center treated dozens of burns on young children who came into contact with these hot stoves. To remedy this problem, the Environmental Health Division constructed barriers around the stoves in shacks throughout the county to prevent burns. (Photo courtesy of Dan Bernstein, Southern Historical Collection, University of North Carolina at Chapel Hill).

The condition of people's homes was yet another obstacle to James and his team in improving health conditions, because the run-down condition of the shacks was often a health hazard in its own right. "I would say about 65 to 70 percent of the housing in that entire area for black folk would simply be unfit for human habitation," James reported. In addition to seeing homes invaded by vermin, the health center regularly saw patients injured from falls through broken planks or off of porches without stairs. One of the most dangerous health hazards in many of these plantation shacks was a metal stove, which was usually the only means of heating the home. The first winter that the health center was opened, Geiger's staff saw dozens of burned children, which took them by surprise. Then they found the reason: "People had tin stoves in the middle of their shacks," Geiger said. "The kids were cold and got up next to it and their clothing caught on fire." In response, the environmental health team designed and installed fences around these stoves to protect children from getting too close, and the burns stopped.[24]

Housing soon became a centerpiece of James's program for environmental health in the Delta. "We are involved in housing because it is closely linked to medical crisis," he said. At one point the Environmental Health Team had a fifteen-man construction crew that traveled throughout north Bolivar County, building stairs and porches; patching walls, floors, and roofs; screening in doors and windows. James and Geiger saw this work as preventative medicine, and fought for OEO funds to improve housing in the name of good health. It was often a frustrating battle for James, as the extreme poverty of his clients regularly undid his good work. "Often we would go out the next spring and we will have to put those same planks back because in the winter the person can't get fuel for his fire so he'll simply use the material that is in his home," he recalled. "People themselves will just take the planks off themselves and burn them."[25]

As with many of the programs James initiated, local whites stood in opposition. "We have to overcome the hostilities of the white plantation owner if we want to work with the black tenants . . . and you have to deal in such a way that, to him, we are not really trying to cause social change," James said in an interview. He recalled visiting one woman living on a local plantation who had a history of miscarriages. "When we went out to look at her house, I could understand why, because there was no stoop to the house—she had to jump up and down off the step." Because her house was owned by the plantation owner, James had to get his permission before building a new set of steps. "I had told him what was going on and he was a little bit not too amicable at first, and then I heard this voice in the back, who . . . said, 'Oh dad, let the man build the steps for Sadie, you know they've been with us for 30 years.'"[26]

Beyond the difficulties encountered from white landowners, James also often had problems convincing black residents that he and his team were there to help them, as most county residents did not see the connections between health and environment. "You have to offer something" to get into their house, James said. "Even if they assist us in doing it, they have to feel that they are going to come out with something

[24] Interview with Andy James, Delta Health Center Tapes; Interview with H. Jack Geiger by Robert Korstad and Neil Boothby.

[25] Interview with Andy James, Delta Health Center Tapes; Howard, "Report of a Work Project in the Environmental Services Division of Tufts–Delta Health Center, 11.

[26] Interview with Andy James, Delta Health Center Tapes; Andy James interviewed by Tom Ward.

more than we did." Insect control was one of the main avenues that James used to build trust with local residents. He did not have to convince residents of the health benefits of insect control, he only had to convince them that he was going to alleviate the nuisance of the bugs. "Often we get into the community by offering some pesticide skills in applying this stuff," he recalled. "If we can get inside the home and we apply the pesticides, and . . . correct the conditions that these pests will flourish under, then maybe we can really get to work with that family. It's a great thing for them. It's a great thing for us, too, in terms of disease control. But it's an even better mechanism for getting into a tough community."[27]

James and his team also relied on the health center's physicians and public health nurses to identify homes across the area that needed their services. Thelma Walker was the head of nursing at the Tufts–Delta Health Center in the late 1960s. "If a nurse in the field finds a home without a water supply—some families have carried every drop for miles all their lives, some have scraped the scum off ditches and use the water underneath—out go the engineers with the well digger invented right here at the center and they dig a well in half a day," she recalled. "If there are rats coming through the floor, we exterminate them. A leaking roof? A privy falling down? Out go workers from the center—and these are local people—to patch the roof, build a new privy or take . . . tools from the tool bank we've scrounged together so they can make their own repairs." Environmental services also worked closely with the health center's public health nurses through its "Acute Home Care Package." Because of the lack of hospital space in the region, or to deal with an issue of short-term acute illness, at the request of the health center's medical staff the environmental team would deliver to someone's home a chemical commode, chlorinated water supply, a portable hospital bed, and portable washing machine for their use until they recovered. By 1971 the Acute Home Care Package reached 400 homes a year in north Bolivar County.[28]

Just as the Tufts–Delta Health Center took a broad view of what encompassed health care, the Environmental Health Services Division took a similarly broad view of what encompassed environmental health. Besides working on issues like clean water, vector control, and home repairs, the environmental team worked with other members of the Tufts–Delta Health Center to provide a host of programs on home economics in order to help community members, most of whom had limited education and finances, make the most of their scarce material resources. To this end, classes were offered on how to use, mend, and remake clothes; hints on meal planning; help for new mothers on how to manage their time; instruction on food preparation and sewing; and help on budgeting so that families could save up enough to purchase

[27] Interview with Andy James, Delta Health Center Tapes.
[28] Kelley, "Health Care in the Mississippi Delta"; Geiger, "A Health Center for Social Change."

(usually secondhand) appliances such as commodes, vaporizers, and refrigerators. The health center even loaned sewing machines and washing machines to needy residents.[29]

Geiger and James were able to sustain OEO funding for the center's variety of environmental health programs by citing simple economics. "We have been able to convince OEO that it is near criminal to consider a comprehensive health service center able to provide such care with a defective environmental base," wrote James. The OEO agreed to fund what became known as the "Basic Sanitation Package," which provided up to $200 worth of services for needy households. The package consisted of a driven well with a hand pump for water, the installation of a sanitary pit privy, screening of doors and windows, the patching of leaky roofs, and the repair of dangerous floors, walls, and stairs. By 1971, the Environmental Health Services Division was installing two hundred Basic Sanitation Packages per year. "It cost seventy-five bucks to dig a well and about the same to build a privy with local labor. Hospitalization in those years cost $600," recalled Geiger. "So we got funded."[30]

* * *

In 1969 Andrew James was the only black sanitarian in the state of Mississippi, a condition that he actively sought to change by bringing more locals into the profession during his time in Mound Bayou. "Training is the lifeblood of this [health] center," James told one interviewer. "What we are trying to do is train young people, young blacks, to introduce them to new disciplines in life."[31] James recruited local blacks to join his staff—many were ex-teachers with some science background—and discussed the opportunities that environmental health presented. In 1969 James helped secure scholarships for two local residents to study environmental health engineering at the University of Cincinnati and the University of Wisconsin, and in January 1970, he initiated a sanitarian intern program at the Tufts–Delta Health Center. The intern program was part of a reciprocal agreement with Tufts University in which engineering students from Tufts would participate in environmental health work in Bolivar County for six months; qualified interns from Mound Bayou would, in turn, be able to enroll in the engineering curriculum at Tufts. James created the curriculum and invited guest sanitarians from across the country to come to Mound Bayou to lecture. The internship program introduced students to the basics of environmental science in order to prepare them to pass a national exam administered by the National Association of Sanitarians. Students

---

[29] Comprehensive Health Services Career Development Technical Assistance Bulletin," Vol. 1, No. 10, Dec. 1970 in Box 20, Folder 145, *DHC*.

[30] James, "The Organization of an Environmental Health Unit...."; Howard, S. J., "Report of a Work Project in the Environmental Services Division of Tufts–Delta Health Center"; Geiger, "A Health Center for Social Change"; Interview with H. Jack Geiger by Robert Korstad and Neil Boothby.

[31] Interview with Andy James, Delta Health Center Tapes.

could take this exam after passing the course at the health center and taking the required college-level science and math courses to satisfy the national requirements.[32]

The initial intern program attracted six local students, all of whom were in their twenties and employed in the Environmental Services Division at the time. The program was demanding: Students took introductory classes in math, chemistry, and biology, and then went on to advanced classes in microbiology, epidemiology, water and wastewater sanitation, laboratory analysis of water, chlorination of water supplies, solid waste disposal, genetics, pesticides, basic elements of surveying, milk and food sanitation, and radiological health. They also took field trips to sanitary landfills, water and wastewater treatment facilities, restaurants, meatpacking plants, and dairy farms. Paul Francis Howard, a graduate student at Tufts who worked at the health center and taught a number of the classes in the program, recalled that

> The extremely heavy workload imposed on these working students forced them to become, in reality, studying workers. . . . There were three two-hour classes each week, scheduled during the afternoon. The responsibilities of the sanitarian students' work sometimes prohibited their attendance at class, and at other times caused them to be distracted or exhausted. . . . Most of the other courses offered at the Health Center met at night, but night classes would have virtually eliminated the Sanitarian Intern Program because most of the students had to work at other jobs at night in order to support their wives and children.[33]

Of this initial group, Charles Washington was the first to successfully complete the program. In February 1971 he enrolled in the graduate program in environmental health engineering at Tufts University, becoming the first member of the environmental health intern program to participate in the educational exchange program with Tufts; he later became the first registered sanitarian to emerge from the program. Eventually, a dozen Bolivar County students would complete the sanitarian intern program at Tufts–Delta Health Center, earn their advanced degrees, and return to Mississippi—the first licensed black sanitarians in the state's history (after Andrew James). The success of this program, according to John Hatch, "was due in large measure to the vision and diplomatic skills of Andy James, coupled

---

[32] Andrew James, "Tufts–Delta Administers Environmental Treatment," *The Journal of Environmental Health*, Vol. 31, No. 5 (March-April, 1969): 437–46; Howard, "Report of a Work Project in the Environmental Services Division of Tufts–Delta Health Center," 78–81.

[33] Howard, "Report of a Work Project in the Environmental Services Division of Tufts–Delta Health Center, Mound Bayou, Mississippi," 78–81.

with generous responses from his friends [at the] University of Cincinnati, Tufts University, and the National Association of Sanitarians." James's intern program, according to Hatch, "[built] nontraditional pathways to opportunity" for young African Americans in the Delta and "stimulated . . . awareness of the burden of neglect placed on poor, rural Americans." As a result of the success of the program, health centers throughout the South began sending their staff to Mound Bayou for environmental training, which led to the establishment of environmental health units at rural health centers in South Carolina, North Carolina, Arkansas, and Virginia.[34] The desire to train local residents to become sanitarians was a major goal of Andy James, and became perhaps his greatest legacy.

In 1971, at a time when the health center was undergoing dramatic changes with its leadership that would drastically alter its mission and programs, Andrew James left Mound Bayou to pursue graduate studies. At that time, many of the health center's most innovative programs, especially those within its Environmental Health Division—like home repair, well drilling, and education—which did not fit a traditional concept of what "health care" entailed, were cut, as they were no longer viewed as a vital part of health care delivery by the federal government. In an attempt to preserve funding for environmental health programs at the Delta Health Center, in late-1971, David Weeks, then director of the center, testified before the Senate Committee on Nutrition and Human Needs:

> I believe profoundly that it is a waste of time, a cynical revolving door, unless "health" also means doing something about the water supply, about sewage, about housing, about food; unless we find a way to deliver integrated health services . . . to whole communities; unless we find a way, far beyond the limits of what is originally meant by "preventative medicine," to go after the social, environmental and economic roots of rural poverty and ill health.[35]

Weeks's pleas, however, fell on deaf ears, and funding for most of the environmental and educational programs at the Delta Health Center was soon eliminated. As early as 1973, Herman Johnson, a Mound Bayou alderman and patient coordinator at the health center, lamented that the impact on the community could already be felt:

> We were concerned with water and sanitation, with helping people build better homes, with creating better living conditions for people. We were battling

---

[34] Howard, "Report of a Work Project in the Environmental Services Division of Tufts–Delta Health Center," 78–81; Hatch narrative, *JHC*.

[35] C. G. McDaniel, "Community Health Centers More Than Clinics for the Poor," *Arizona Republic*, Sept. 5, 1971.

disease at its source. Now we're back to treating the results of bad environmental conditions that will just continue to produce the same health problems in the same people over and over again.[36]

The case of the Tufts–Delta Health Center's Environmental Health Services programs provides an interesting microcosm of the War on Poverty as a whole. The environmental programs of the Tufts–Delta Health Center were broad-based, creative, and fairly expensive. They also were given very little time to succeed before they were financially cut off at the knees and their leadership was overhauled. There can be very little argument that the work done by Andy James's Environmental Health Unit was both needed and successful in improving the health of residents of north Bolivar County–and that the loss of these environmental services negatively affected the quality of life of Bolivar County's poor. Although some of the programs initiated by Andy James during his tenure at the Tufts–Delta Health Center, most notably the fight for sewage systems for all residents of Bolivar County, were eventually undertaken by local governments, many of the other services simply died away with the loss of the Environmental Health Unit. Twenty years after the founding of Tufts–Delta Health Center, eighteen Delta counties still faced water shortages and/or unsafe water sources. In 1988, 11 percent of northern Bolivar County's population still lacked complete plumbing, and 60 percent of the families still had no wells.[37] Any honest evaluation of the Tufts–Delta Health Center (and, in many ways, many War on Poverty projects as a whole) needs to take into account what it had achieved, and was achieving, at the time that it saw its funding gutted. In many ways the perceived failure of the Great Society was ensured by those who cut off the financial lifeblood of its programs.

---

[36] Huttie, "New Federalism and the Death of a Dream in Mound Bayou, Mississippi," 29.

[37] L. C. Dorsey. "Dirt Dauber Nest, Socks Nailed Over Doorways, Salts, Prayer, and OTC's: Space Age Medicine in the Poor Community," Unpublished manuscript, *DHC*.

We started this farm with nothing. We didn't have a hoe. We didn't have a tractor.
We didn't have a plow. We didn't have anything. We had to depend on black farmers
around for tools and land.

WILLIE FINCH[1]

The land was here; the people were here; and the hunger was here.

L.C. DORSEY[2]

5

The Farm Co-op

AS JOHN HATCH traveled through north Bolivar County in 1966 and 1967, drumming up support for the health center and organizing the local health associations, he repeatedly ran into people such as the mother who told him, "It is nice to learn about health, but I think maybe if you could find us work so we can get enough to eat, there would be a better chance of us having good health."[3] Hunger was the most pressing problem facing north Bolivar County's black poor in the mid-1960s, and although the food prescriptions introduced at the Tufts–Delta Health Center provided needed relief to the malnourished population of the county, they were by no means a solution to the chronic hunger in the region. Geiger and Hatch realized that the ability of the center's physicians and nurses to deliver adequate health care would be rendered moot if the diets of people in the center's target populations could not be improved.

The problem of hunger in Mississippi's Delta region was already acute by the time the Tufts–Delta Health Center opened its doors for patients in 1967. At the time, 470,000 Mississippians received food stamps—roughly 10 percent of the national total—but due to the rising entry costs of the program, many more poor blacks

---

[1] Black, *People and Plows Against Hunger,* x.
[2] L. C. Dorsey interviewed by Robert Korstad and Neil Boothby, April 22, 1992, Southern Rural Poverty Collection http://dewitt.sanford.duke.edu/wp-content/uploads/2011/09/DORSEY1.pdf
[3] James, "Tufts–Delta Administers Environmental Treatment," 444.

in the Delta could not afford them. Indeed, a 1967 U.S. Civil Rights Commission study found that eight Mississippi counties that had switched from commodity distribution to food stamps experienced a decrease of almost 36,000 poor people receiving food aid.[4]

Further exacerbating the state's food-stamp inequities was the fact that the program was controlled by the state's white power structure. The U.S. Civil Rights Commission found that the state's Department of Welfare, which administered the program, was in violation of the Civil Rights Act of 1964 in its management of the food stamp program, resulting in many black Mississippians either not receiving as much aid as they were eligible for or being improperly denied aid outright. A Jesuit seminarian, Paul Francis Howard, who spent a number of months working at the Tufts–Delta Health Center, observed, "Questionable accounting methods are used in figuring the amount of food stamps for which a family is eligible, and inappropriate guidelines have been established which fail to acknowledge the real needs of many Blacks in the area. Some of the supermarkets take advantage of the Food Stamp Program by raising their prices when Food Stamps are issued."[5]

In the face of this challenge, Jack Geiger again looked to his experiences in South Africa with Sidney and Emily Kark for inspiration. The Karks had established a community vegetable garden near the Pholela Health Center where members of the local population could supplement their meager diets. Children picked vegetables for their midday meal, and expectant mothers received "take-home packages" in order to improve prenatal health. Because of demand, the Pholela center's vegetable program soon expanded. Schools installed their own gardens, and students grew, harvested, and prepared their daily meals. Home vegetable gardens also were developed with the aid of the center, as people were taught how to cultivate a variety of vegetables that greatly improved their diets, and, subsequently, their overall health. As home vegetable gardens became more common in the township, small cooperatives were established for residents to purchase seeds and tools, and eventually a market was established at the health center for people to sell and trade their produce and other homemade goods.[6]

[4] "Materials on Hunger," Folder 15, Lee Bankhead Papers, Wisconsin Historical Society Archives, Madison, Wisc.; Alice Sardell, *The U.S. Experiment in Social Medicine: The Community Health Center Program, 1965–1986* (Pittsburgh, Pa.: University of Pittsburg Press, 1988): 209; Marian Wright Edelman, "Still Hungry in America," *The Huffington Post*, Feb. 2, 2102 (http://www.huffingtonpost.com/marian-wright-edelman/hunger-in-america_b_1269450.html#es_share_ended).

[5] "Materials on Hunger," Folder 15, Lee Bankhead Papers; Howard, "Report of a Work Project in the Environmental Services Division of Tufts–Delta Health Center," 92–93.

[6] Kark, *Promoting Community Health*, 39, 50–52.

Geiger asked whether a similar program could work in the Mississippi Delta. The soil was some of the richest in the world, and almost all of the people most in need of food had at least some farming experience. He met with John Hatch and Roy Brown, a physician and nutritionist at the Tufts–Delta Health Center, to try to come up with a plan. Their initial idea was to help the people of north Bolivar County cultivate small plots of land in and around the plantation shacks where so many of them lived. The health center would provide seeds and tools, and the people could grow family gardens to supplement their diets.

It soon became apparent that small family gardens would not be practical for a number of reasons. First, any land that tenants had access to was owned by someone else, someone who usually was unwilling to turn over any of it for family gardens. Even if the tenants were granted some land to cultivate on their own, it would usually be right next to the cotton rows, which were regularly sprayed by herbicides and insecticides that would contaminate the vegetables.[7]

Hatch then put forth the idea of a community garden, "a plot of maybe a couple of acres where people could come and grow stuff." He asked Brown about what types of foods would be easy to grow in the Delta, which people would eat, and that packed a nutritional punch. Brown recommended southern peas and okra, both of which were high in vegetable protein and already staples of the Southern diet. Hatch then took his idea for a community garden to the local health associations, to see whether there was any interest. "We thought we would get fifty or sixty people," recalled Geiger, "and about a thousand families raised their hands." Hatch decided that if there was that kind of interest, and so many people with agricultural skills, they should try to get some funding to rent or buy a large tract of land, grow food instead of cotton, and create a farm cooperative for the poor people of north Bolivar County. "It was clear," he recalled, "that searching for a way to produce and control food was more exciting for many people than healthcare. While nutrition was vitally important to health, it was not regarded as a health intervention. People were confident about their ability to feed themselves if they had access to land and equipment."[8]

Cooperative farms in the Mississippi Delta existed as far back as the 1930s, and there were attempts throughout the region to develop new cooperatives during the civil rights era. Bolivar County itself had been the site of one of the most controversial farm co-ops in the state: the interracial Delta Cooperative Farm, founded by members of the Southern Tenant Farmers Union (STFU) in 1934 near Hillhouse.

---

[7] Ward interview with Geiger and Hatch; Black, *People and Plows*, 5.
[8] Ward interview with Geiger and Hatch; Korstad and Boothby interview with H. Jack Geiger; John Hatch narrative, *JHC*.

The 2,000-acre farm was supported by Northern philanthropists and settled by eighteen black and twelve white families. Members built their own houses, established a general store, operated a school, and even had a health clinic. The co-op was governed by a five-person council drawn from the member families; no more than three members of the council could be of one race. Although theologian Reinhold Niebuhr—one of the cooperative's financial backers—labeled the project "the most significant experiment in social Christianity now being conducted in America," many of the activities on the farm were strictly segregated, in an attempt not to rouse too much white hostility to the project. Despite the segregation of most of the farm's arrangements, local white ire for the cooperative was raised by both the education of black children, including many who came to the cooperative school from neighboring plantations, and the practice of all the members, black and white, to use courtesy titles to refer to one another. Eventually, the combination of these external pressures and internal strife led to the dissolution of the Delta Cooperative Farm in 1941.[9]

In neighboring Washington County, an organization called "Freedom City" was established in 1966 on 400 acres southeast of Greenville. Based on the model of an Israeli *kibbutz*, it sought to provide an alternative to black migration to Northern cities for sharecroppers displaced by mechanization. Aided by the Delta Ministry, the largest civil rights organization in Mississippi, and funded by both the Office of Economic Opportunity (OEO) and the Ford Foundation, Freedom City sought to provide vocational training for the displaced sharecroppers and to develop a self-sustaining farming and industrial cooperative. Twenty-two families moved into prefabricated homes (with no running water, electricity, or heat) erected on the site. Although the families lived separately, they cooked and ate communally in a large farmhouse that came with the land. Beset with difficulties from the start, plans for the eventual construction of fifty permanent homes were never realized (only twenty were built), and the cooperative struggled to find markets for its agricultural goods or attract industrial development. Federal funds for the program were eliminated in the early 1970s, and residents began to move out.[10]

Hatch's plan was less ambitious than that of Freedom City; he wanted only to focus on providing food to the hungry. "We were trying to set up a way for people to use the skills that they already had," Hatch stated, "to solve what was really their number one health problem, which was nutrition." Although initial enthusiasm for the project was substantial, the task was overwhelming. "When community health

[9] Asch, *The Senator & the Sharecropper*, 87; Neil R. McMillen, *Dark Journey: Black Mississippians in the Age of Jim Crow* (Urbana and Chicago: University of Illinois Press, 1989): 24, 94.
[10] Newman, *Divine Agitators*, 127–148.

organizers reported the names of over 300 families interested in gardening, I knew we had a problem," he remembered. The number of families "exceeded the scale of common family gardening. . . . I had grown up on a farm, but I was way over my head and I knew it."[11]

For counsel, Hatch called on his cousin Rupert Seals, a professor of agriculture at the University of Iowa. Seals said that the smaller-scale farming Hatch was considering was common in the 1920s and 1930s, but had been displaced by rising demand and improved technology in the 1940s and 1950s. "John," he said, "I can tell you how to do a million pounds, but damn if I know how to do five thousand." Seals recommended that Hatch contact Professor Robert Woodruff at the University of Georgia, who was an expert in smaller-scale production technology of the 1920s and 1930s. Hatch did, and from there on both Seals and Woodruff became unpaid consultants, advisors, and facilitators to the project. Both visited Mound Bayou to gain hands-on practice and insight toward a more thorough understanding of the challenge of the farm cooperative.[12]

On December 9, 1967, Hatch chaired a meeting for sixty-four community representatives about developing the farm cooperative. At that time, the co-op still had no land, tools, or funding. Isaac Daniels, a local black farmer, agreed to donate ten acres of his land near Mound Bayou to the project, and others soon stood up to offer tools and seed. Over the subsequent weeks, Hatch scrambled to try to acquire more land and supplies, and to organize the volunteers. Friends of Geiger donated two new Ford tractors, and organizers were ready to plant in the spring of 1968. By then, Hatch had procured 128 acres of land for the co-op to farm, much of it loaned or leased from the county's more prosperous black farmers. He had signed up over 500 families, at fifty cents each, as co-op members. Throughout the county, people wanted to participate in the "big garden," as many called it, by either working in the fields or buying its produce. Membership in the co-op was initially restricted to households earning less than $1,000 a year, and all members who were able worked the fields, earning $4 a day in cash and $6 a day in produce. The poorest families— those with household incomes less than $200 per person—were given the first opportunities to work on the farm.[13]

Once there were seeds in the ground for the first crop, Hatch began securing funding to allow the co-op to expand and thrive. He first approached Tufts University, which provided $5,000 for seed and tools, and donated twelve acres of land it

---

[11] Ward interview with Geiger and Hatch.

[12] John Hatch narrative, *JHC*.

[13] Black, *People and Plows*, 6–7: L. C. Dorsey, "North Bolivar County Farm Cooperative, A. A. L. 1969 Progress Report," in John Hatch Papers, Southern Historical Collection, UNC–Chapel Hill (hereafter *JHP*); North Bolivar County Farm Co-op Minutes, August 2, 1968, in Box 118, Folder 875, *DHC*.

had bought for the health center but decided would not be needed. A Madison, Wisconsin, civil rights group, Measure for Measure, donated $10,000 to the co-op, which provided the down payment for the co-op's first land purchase. Geiger and Hatch then turned to OEO, writing a $152,000 proposal for what they carefully titled a "nutritional demonstration grant," in order to avoid any controversy that critics might arouse regarding the farm being some sort of communist program. In the proposal, they argued that on the farm "agriculturally oriented rural, poor families can grow most of the food necessary for reasonable maintenance of themselves," instead of going on the dole, and that the project would help the participants acquire "(a) skills and management; (b) increased understanding of the relationship of diet to good health; and (c) heightened self-esteem." The OEO agreed to fund the "nutritional demonstration" grant, as long as it was administered by Tufts University; Tufts officials agreed, and the funding was approved on May 1, 1968. Leaders of the Tufts–Delta Health Center also approached the Ford Foundation for support of the farm, which eventually resulted in funding for the co-op to purchase an additional 300 acres of land. The hope was that with federal and foundation support, the co-op could become self-sustaining in three years.[14]

Hatch then contacted the agricultural department at Mississippi State University and developed a relationship with the faculty there to provide guidance on how to develop the cooperative farm. He found that the faculty there were excited about the opportunity to work with the co-op. Geiger remembers that the faculty at Mississippi State "were so intrigued by the idea that the Delta might diversify into vegetable gardening, instead of just cotton and soybeans, that they sent a senior consultant to work with the farm manager, both to lend technical advice and to study the project." Dr. Harrell Hammit and Dr. Gale Ammerman made the 280-mile round trip from Starkville to Mound Bayou three or four times a month to help educate the co-op workers on how to transition from cotton farming to vegetable production. They instructed co-op members in horticultural methods for growing vegetables, knowledge which few people in the Mississippi Delta had, even though they had grown up on farms. Hatch was surprised, however, to find that not everyone in the black community was happy with his decision to reach out to Mississippi State University, which had only admitted its first African-American student, Richard Holmes, in 1965. "I was criticized a lot for cooperating with the white folk and all that kind of stuff," he recalled, but "that's where the resources were." He told people, "I'm not going to sit up here and question this man about his position on civil rights

---

[14] John Hatch narrative, *JHC*; Black, *People and Plows*, 26–27; Finney and David McGranahan, "Community Support and Goal Displacement in a Poor Peoples' Cooperative Farm," 13–14, *DHC*; Notes, Folder 10, Lee Bankhead Papers; "What is Measure for Measure?" Folder 14, Lee Bankhead papers.

if I think I can get some support or technical assistance from him that we need. . . . If I want somebody to give me a technical opinion on how to grow peas, or grow greens, or keep down the bugs, I don't need to know his position on civil rights." Hatch's willingness to engage local whites—as well as his success in garnering their support—for the farm cooperative and other health center programs, proved to be one of his great talents, and was crucial to the early success of the program.[15]

In addition to assistance from Mississippi State, Hatch also received support from a number of local white leaders for the co-op. Because they controlled the needed agricultural resources in the Delta, Hatch knew that it would be necessary to engage some of the large planters if the co-op was going to succeed. "I had assumed that most people were decent," Hatch recalled. "They might be racist, but they don't want to see kids hungry and people starving," so he believed he could get their support for the farm co-op. His optimism was rewarded with the response that he received from a number of local whites. For example, Hatch went to the Stovall Plantation in neighboring Coahoma County to buy a ton of potatoes to plant. When Mr. Stovall asked what he intended to do with the potatoes, Hatch explained the co-op to him. Stovall then asked, "How you going to plant 'em?" Hatch replied, "We're going to drop them." Stovall said, "You can't do it that way," and told Hatch that he needed a potato planter. Hatch, who had never seen a potato planter, was discouraged, until Stovall told him, "Now I've got a cutter and a planter here. . . . Just take it immediately. If it is useful you can pay me." Hatch left the plantation that day with the potato planter, recalling that "we eventually paid him . . . $300 or something."[16]

Another unlikely white supporter of the co-op was the president of the Mississippi Chemical Cooperative (MCC), Owen Cooper. When Hatch inquired about purchasing fertilizer for the farm cooperative, Cooper responded that the MCC's pricing models would not suit Hatch's needs: the majority of Cooper's buyers were plantation owners who owned stock in the chemical cooperative, allowing them to pay a certain amount when they bought the fertilizer, then later receive a rebate up to 20 percent depending on their profits and losses. Such a system, while beneficial for members who paid the $10,000 membership fee, made it difficult for a small operation like the farm co-op to purchase goods at an affordable price. Hatch was discouraged until Cooper made him an offer: "I think what you are trying to do over there is worthwhile, and I'm going to treat you as if you were a stockholder"— in essence, allow Hatch gratis membership in the chemical cooperative, granting

[15] Sobelson, "Participation, Power, and Place," 70; Black, *People and Plows*, 27; H. Y. Ward interviewed by John Hatch.

[16] H. Y. Ward interviewed by John Hatch; Ward interview with Geiger and Hatch.

him discounted access to fertilizer, fuel, and seed in the years that followed. Hatch described this offer as "an act of high decency" that gave the farm co-op a chance to succeed.[17]

Geiger and Hatch were delighted with the support they received from select people throughout the Delta—black and white—who wanted to see the project succeed. "The idea of people attempting to help themselves revealed many submerged resources," Hatch later wrote. A white planter loaned the co-op needed farm machinery and arranged for his employees to teach the men how to operate it. Several black and white farmers allowed their employees to volunteer their time to the co-op and provided equipment and fuel to help out after regular working hours. "Through the donations that we were able to get," Hatch wrote, "we purchased seed and rented tractors from local farmers, sometimes driving them at night, on Saturdays and Sundays, just to make certain that we had some type of crop planted." Members of the professional staff at the health center came out and worked in the fields after hours and on weekends. Chris Hansen remembered that he and his wife "picked collard greens, black-eyed peas, and sweet potatoes with our children. . . . We did it to show solidarity, but our neighbors worked there to provide for their basic survival needs."[18]

Although many people were excited about the co-op, Hatch encountered difficulty in cases where potential members feared that joining the co-op would make them ineligible for welfare benefits or would elicit retribution from their white landlords and employers—or both. Black fear of white reprisal—especially economic reprisal—remained a very real obstacle for organizers of both the health center and the co-op, even in the late 1960s. A number of black church leaders, whom Hatch had counted on to be advocates for the co-op, counseled their parishioners against becoming members. Some preachers feared they would have to compete with the co-op for the time and limited funds of their parishioners. "There was opposition from [the more privileged] white folk and black folk [to the co-op]," recalled Hatch. "They were saying, 'You know, we love these [poor] folk, but you should not spend so much time [on them] because they just don't have a notion of the modern world or all this stuff you are talking about.'" Much of the opposition centered on the very idea of a co-op, and Geiger noted that in order to deflect some of the opposition for the farm cooperative, "which sounds suspiciously communistic in the Mississippi environment," he made sure to refer to it instead as a "nutrition demonstration

---

[17] H. Y. Ward interviewed by John Hatch; Ward interview with Geiger and Hatch.

[18] John Hatch narrative, *JHP*; John Hatch, "Historical Sketch and Progress Report on the North Bolivar County Farm Cooperative," (January 1969), in Folder 10, Lee Bankhead Papers; Hansen, *In the Name of the Children*, 72–73.

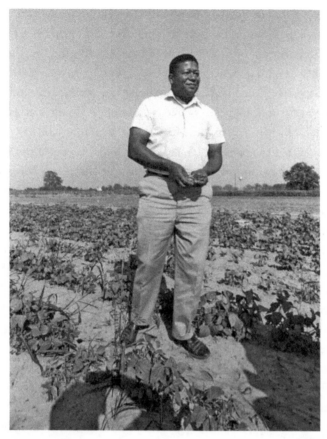

FIGURE 5.1 John Hatch at the Co-op Farm (Photo courtesy of Dan Bernstein, Southern Historical Collection, University of North Carolina at Chapel Hill).

project" rather than a co-op, especially when asking for funding. "That sanction, the umbrella of health, made an enormous difference," he believed.[19]

The work on the co-op also took Hatch away from his duties with the health center. "At times, it seemed as [if the] movement toward food security would overwhelm and compromise the effort toward bringing the health council into existence," he remembered. "The Office of Economic Opportunity demanded a health council and wondered why it was taking so long," but he believed that "the people we came to serve placed higher priority on food security," and so he was committed to getting the co-op off the ground. He had never intended the co-op to be an appendage of the Tufts–Delta Health Center, but instead envisioned a cooperative farm owned and run by the poor people themselves. Throughout 1968 Hatch worked to organize

[19] Black, *People and Plows*, 8; Ward interview with Hatch and Geiger; Interview with Geiger by Korstad and Boothby.

a dozen "co-op clubs" throughout the county to serve, in many ways, like the local health associations. Committees were set up in each club to manage recruitment of members, transportation of workers, and distribution of produce. The co-op clubs then established a board of directors, made up of two representatives from each club, to run the cooperative, and hired a farm manager and a project director.[20]

To run the farm, the newly incorporated North Bolivar County Farm Cooperative's board hired John Brown, a thirty-nine-year-old father of nine who had only a fourth-grade education. For the previous ten years Brown had managed the 446-acre soybean and cotton plantation of Abe Miller in nearby Gunnison, Mississippi, where he oversaw eighteen workers. Brown had helped organize the health associations in Gunnison and Perthshire and was one of the earliest supporters of the farm co-op. "When Mr. Hatch first tried to get me come here and work for the black man's welfare, I had a terrible time making up my mind," Brown recalled. "It worried me sick. I was doing pretty good—not making much salary, mind you, but enough to feed my wife and nine children." He was convinced, however, that the co-op was "a great idea of giving people, training young people, to work. . . . And so we decided to make our home over there, and we're still trying to get it done and train the young people how to work—keep them from sitting up there waiting on the welfare check, or some other kind of check like that. . . . Learn them how to do the work and stand up on their own two feet." Brown was elected to the position by the co-op's board, which paid him $180 a month to run the farm, where he was charged with overseeing the property's production of mustard greens, collard greens, okra, onions, lima beans, black powder beans, sweet potatoes, white potatoes, and Mississippi silver peas. He told *LIFE* magazine's Richard Hall, "Working here for this co-op is just broad daylight in my life."[21]

John Hatch was elected the co-op's first project director, but he soon had to resign the position because of his duties at the health center. In a tremendous surprise to Hatch, the co-op's board elected to replace him with L. C. Dorsey, a 29-year-old civil rights activist and mother of six who had recently been hired to an entry-level position as a training associate and outreach worker at the Tufts–Delta Health Center. Dorsey would go on to become one of the health center's most important figures. In her position at the health center, she helped recruit people from the surrounding communities to be trained as nurses' aides and environmental aides. She also

[20] John Hatch narrative, *JHC*; Henry C. Finney and David McGranahan, "Community Support and Goal Displacement in a Poor Peoples' Cooperative Farm: A Case Study of Organizational Adaptation to Environmental Uncertainty," paper presented at the Rural Sociological Society, August 26, 1972, Box 119, Folder 886, *DHC*.

[21] Interview with John Brown by John Hatch. Southern Historical Collection, UNC–Chapel Hill; L. C. Dorsey Interview, Delta Health Center Tapes (Disk 1, Reel 5-1); John Hatch narrative, *JHC*; Hall, "A Stir of Hope in Mound Bayou," 78; Black, *People and Plows*, 27–28.

traveled the county, garnering local support, first for the health center and then the farm co-op, helping to define community needs.

Hatch initially was disappointed with the board's selection of Dorsey, both because of what he perceived as her inexperience and the fact that the two did not get along on a personal level. "I asked several friends why they had seen fit to select a young woman to a demanding job providing oversight of farming," he recalled. "Several male members had experience as foremen on Delta plantations. I was told that L. C. was smart and hard-working and could bring people together and had done farm work all of her life. Over time, I could see the wisdom of their choice."[22]

L. C. Dorsey knew farming, and she knew poverty. Born in 1938 in Tribbett, the daughter of Mississippi sharecroppers, she grew up on Delta plantations. Dorsey began working in the cotton fields at age eight, and dropped out of high school at seventeen when she became pregnant and married a son of sharecroppers from a neighboring plantation. She gave birth to six children across eight pregnancies over a span of ten years and seemed destined to the life of poverty and lack of opportunity that ensnarled most black Mississippians during the mid-twentieth century. As mechanization and chemicals changed cotton agriculture in the region, Dorsey, then pregnant with her sixth child, and her husband were put off the plantation they were living on and moved into a three-room shotgun home in Shelby. "In many ways our condition of poverty was downgraded," she recalled. "On the farm, we lived in a house rent-free, and the part-time work paid 30 to 50 cents per hour. We had wood for heating and we had someone to borrow money from for food, utilities and for a visit to the doctor. Being kicked off the plantation meant that we were on our own for all of our living expenses: rent, utilities, food, and health care."[23]

In Shelby, Dorsey's husband found a job working for a lumber company for $36 a week. Unable to find a job in town, Dorsey sought day labor, working in the fields of local plantations to supplement the family's meager income. She recalled that it "was the first time . . . where I had been totally without food. I had one horrible, nightmarish night where we cooked the last food at noon. . . and we all went to bed that night hungry. . . . We had no money and no food in the house."[24]

Dorsey's life changed when Annie Devine and Victoria Gray of the Freedom Democratic Party knocked on her door. She joined the civil rights movement as a voting rights organizer in the Delta, eventually emerging as one of Fannie Lou Hamer's chief lieutenants in the fight for civil rights in Mississippi. She organized

---

[22] L. C. Dorsey narrative, L. C. Dorsey papers (private, in the possession of the author; hereafter *LCDP*); John Hatch narrative, *JHC*.

[23] L.C. Dorsey, "Dirt Dauber Nest. . ."

[24] Dorsey, *Freedom Came to Mississippi*, 19; Interview with L. C. Dorsey by Robert Korstad and Neil Boothby.

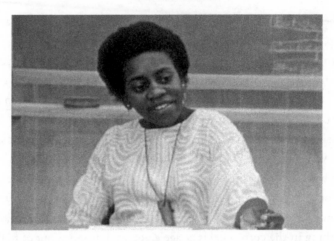

FIGURE 5.2 L. C. Dorsey (Photo Credit: Victor Schoenbach).

boycotts, including the one of Shelby's downtown stores, and voter registration drives throughout the state. While continuing to volunteer for numerous civil rights organizations, in 1966 Dorsey took a job working for Head Start, where she was trained as a teacher. "Head Start offered an opportunity," Dorsey recalled, "and I learned a lot about the organized workplace.... Teaching a classroom had a certain amount of power that I never envisioned, that you never perceive, being a student. And you could impact on the people in that classroom in a very positive way. And I enjoyed it."[25]

Soon after it opened, Dorsey came to the Tufts–Delta Health Center for medical care for her children. "I could not afford to have [my children] examined by the local private physicians," she recalled, so the promise of free health care was very attractive. Like many other poor Delta residents, Dorsey previously had relied on home remedies to treat herself and her family. But she was skeptical. "Who were these people and why would they move to Mound Bayou of all places?" she wondered. "It sounded too good to be true and I really was afraid that we may have been targeted for testing of some new drugs or perhaps being studied for something." Her fears were allayed, however, when she arrived at the center. "I never saw an unsegregated waiting room until I took my own children in 1967 to the Delta Health Center," she remembered. "The first time I was called 'Mrs. Dorsey' was at the health center. It was also the first time I saw health care as a right."[26]

Not long after she first came to the health center with her children, John Hatch reached out to Dorsey to join his staff as a community outreach worker—"to do

[25] Dorsey, *Freedom Came to Mississippi*, 19; Interview with L. C. Dorsey by Robert Korstad and Neil Boothby.
[26] Kay Mills, "Dr. Delta," *Mother Jones* (Jan/Feb 1993); L. C. Dorsey narrative, *LCDP*.

workshops as part of the training program for their staff," Dorsey described it. "And that was heady stuff." While she debated leaving her position at Head Start, she eventually decided to join the Tufts–Delta Health Center because she felt that it "embodied, in a much more compelling way than operation Head Start had, all the things that we talked about in the civil rights movement, of empowering people to take control of their communities." Dorsey joined the Tufts–Delta Health Center's staff in 1967; she would be a central figure there for the next three decades, holding a wide variety of positions, starting as a "training associate" and eventually serving as the center's director from 1988 to 1995.[27]

Despite having recruited Dorsey to work at the center (albeit in a different capacity), John Hatch was dismayed by her election as the farm co-op's new director. "She was confrontational," he said of the diminutive and feisty Dorsey. "She called me an 'Uncle Tom', and she was angry." The animosity between them seemed to be rooted in the fact that Hatch, while black and a native Southerner, was, unlike Dorsey, well-educated and had lived outside the South for a significant period of time. She believed he could not relate to the circumstances of poor blacks in the Delta. Their strategies for bringing about change also put them at odds with each other. Schooled in direct-action tactics, and hardened by the violence of the Freedom Movement in Mississippi, Dorsey was skeptical—even distrustful—of working with whites, no matter how well-intentioned they claimed to be. Hatch, who had not participated as an activist in the civil rights movement, was instead intent on quietly building bridges to improve the lives of the Delta poor. Eventually, the two would develop close professional and personal relationships with each other, but in the summer of 1968, as Hatch trained Dorsey to take over the reins as director of the co-op, they spoke to each other only when necessary. As Dorsey later lamented, "There was so much hostility between us that the year of training never took place." As a result, when she took over full control of the administration of the co-op, she felt that she was "no more prepared for the in-depth responsibilities . . . than I'd been when the board hired me."[28]

Perhaps due to their acrimonious relationship, Hatch transitioned his responsibilities to Dorsey without much in the way of a formal handover or orientation. "John is not possessive about his projects," Dorsey commented in 1970, and "he shoved the co-op onto my shoulders before I was quite ready to start full responsibility to take care of the total administration. [The] result was that I had to call on him

[27] Interview with L. C. Dorsey by Robert Korstad and Neil Boothby; Justin Cardon, "L. C. Dorsey," *Jackson Free Press*, August 26, 2013.

[28] Ward interview with Hatch and Geiger; Black, *People and Plows*, 31–32; Dorsey notes, interview with Theodore H. Howe, May 6, 1970, *LCDP*.

for support." Dorsey likewise ran into difficulties working with farm manager John Brown. According to Herbert Black in his history of the farm co-op, *People and Plows Against Hunger*, while Dorsey initially tried to leave the daily operation of the farm up to Brown, she soon became critical of his planning of crop schedules, record keeping, and equipment maintenance. She also faced sexism from Brown and other men on the farm, which contributed to her struggles. Her conflict with Brown came to a head when she asked the co-op board to replace him with a new farm manager. The board—many of whom were very supportive of Brown—declined.[29]

Despite these early problems, the farm co-op's first year could only be described as a success. By the end of 1968 the co-op had about 156 acres under cultivation, distributing tons of snap beans, butter beans, squash, collard greens, sweet potatoes, Irish potatoes, and southern peas to the needy residents of north Bolivar County. Membership in the farm co-op had been upped to one dollar per family per year, and members were entitled to work the fields to earn both cash and food credits—$4 in cash and $6 in food for a day's labor. About 250 members tilled the soil and harvested the crops on the farm that first season. Local towns with co-op clubs or chapters organized to provide transportation for members on different days so that there would be both enough workers on the farm and so that all members who needed to work for their food would have an opportunity to do so. Co-op members who were not able to work in the fields were able to purchase the farm's produce at sharply reduced prices, such as a pound of butter beans for 15 cents, or a pound of potatoes for 6 cents; those who could neither work the fields nor afford to pay for the vegetables received them for free. Many people who could work on the farm donated their food credits to those who were in greater need than themselves.[30]

One of the practical obstacles that soon emerged was how to distribute the produce effectively. The co-op served members living in a rural, 500-square-mile area, and many of those most in need of its produce often had little access to transportation. Initially, the co-op board set up two food distribution centers and hired two people to work the centers at $10 a day; eventually, there would be a dozen co-op distribution centers established throughout north Bolivar County. The local co-op clubs also organized groups to deliver vegetables to those who lacked transportation or were homebound.[31]

---

[29] Dorsey notes, interview with Theodore H. Howe, May 6, 1970, *LCDP*; Black, *People and Plows*, 34–35.

[30] Henry C. Finney and David McGranahan, "Community Support and Goal Displacement...," 13–14; "Malnutrition Notes," in Folder 10, Lee Bankhead Papers; L. C. Dorsey, "North Bolivar County Farm Cooperative, A. A. L, 1969 Progress Report," *JHP*; Maxwell, "The Ailing Poor"; North Bolivar County Farm Co-op Minutes, August 2, 1968, in Box 118, Folder 875, *DHC*.

[31] North Bolivar County Farm Co-op Minutes, August 2, 1968, *DHC*.

Neither the co-op nor many of its members had effective means of storing their harvested vegetables. The leaders of the co-op responded by coming up with two ideas to deal with the problem of food storage: a frozen-food locker and a cannery. The food locker idea took off almost immediately; in its first year of operation the co-op contracted with a facility in nearby Cleveland, Mississippi, to flash freeze and store its produce for distribution throughout the year. The food locker not only provided a means to freeze and store vegetables, but also had facilities to butcher, freeze, and store meat. The co-op board took advantage of this resource by purchasing meat from wholesalers and local famers (some of whom were members of the co-op), then process-ing it and selling it at cost to its members. Most importantly, the food locker provided an affordable and effective means to preserve and store the co-op's produce for year-round distribution to its members. One member recalled that the frozen food locker had "neckbones, and steaks, and hams—cured ham, fresh ham—turkey wings . . ., southern peas, lima beans, string beans, squash, greens, tomatoes," all available for purchase.[32]

The cannery was more of a challenge. John Hatch approached OEO about fund-ing a small cannery that would be operated by the community and geared primarily toward meeting the needs of the co-op's members, with the possibility that any sur-plus goods might be sold locally. Initially, OEO proposed that the co-op reach out to plants that might be willing to can the farm's produce on a contract basis. "We rejected this [idea]," wrote Hatch. "All our lives all we'd ever been able to do was to harvest the raw material, [and] carry it to the white man for the final processing." Hoping to avoid complications and increased costs that would come with employ-ing a middle man, the board began exploring options for buying or building its own cannery.[33]

Hatch proceeded to write an OEO grant to examine the feasibility of a canning plant. He found that it was difficult to find a cannery that would be the appropri-ate size for the co-op. A small plant, as was initially planned, would be heavily de-pendent on manual labor and not produce enough canned goods to be economi-cally viable. The alternative, a larger cannery, was initially very attractive, given that it would allow the co-op to sell its produce across the South and beyond. The idea seemed to be a natural: with so many native Mississippians and other black Southerners living in Northern ghettoes, it was believed that there was bound to be a significant market for canned "soul food" from home. Hatch believed they had

---

[32] North Bolivar County Farm Co-op Minutes, August 2, 1968, *DHC*; "The Delta Health Center Digest," Box 20, Folder 148, *DHC*; Interview with L. C. Dorsey by Robert Korstad and Neil Boothby; Mrs. Young Oral History. Delta Health Center Tapes, Disk 1, Reel 5-10.

[33] Hatch, "Historical Sketch and Progress Report on the North Bolivar County Farm Cooperative," *DHC*.

stumbled on a huge market opportunity: "If you could market Chinese food and Italian food and Jewish food and Irish food in the grocery stores around the country, why couldn't you market a food aimed primarily at the tastes of black people?" In an effort to codify this market, leaders from the co-op and the Tufts–Delta Health Center reached out to Elijah Muhammed, the leader of the Nation of Islam, to ship goods to northern black communities. They even sought permission from the Minnesota-based Green Giant Company to create a "Jolly Black Giant" label for their produce.[34] Neither inquiry brought any leads, and the cannery—along with the line of co-op foods—never materialized. OEO was reluctant to support a cannery because it had already sunk over $3 million into a similar operation in neighboring Sunflower County, which failed. When co-op leaders appealed to OEO to take over the closed plant, they were denied, because of legal and financial difficulties. The lack of a cannery hampered the ability to distribute and store the food that the farm produced, but it did not deter the farm's operation. The food locker in Cleveland proved to be an effective means of keeping the produce from spoiling, and the co-op board increased the number of food distribution centers throughout the county.[35]

By September of 1969 the co-op had become operationally independent of the health center, administered by former day laborers and sharecroppers from throughout north Bolivar County. A board of thirty-six delegates, representing a dozen clubs with an overall membership of 6,000, determined policy for all the farm cooperative's operations. Each member was an equal owner and had a vote in the decisions of the co-op and populating its Board of Directors. As L. C. Dorsey remarked: "They're poor people, all of them! Every last one of them on the board." The board elected its own chair and officers. Will Finch, a carpenter and former sharecropper from Symonds (and former employee of the health center's Environmental Health Unit), was elected as the co-op board's first chairman. He helped guide it through the process of incorporating, getting a charter, setting up bylaws, and hiring John Brown and L. C. Dorsey. Finch was a deacon in his church and was well-known as someone who helped mediate disputes in the community. "Will Finch was a guy who didn't learn to read until he was about 20," recalled John Hatch, but "he was decent, and people know that. He was a good worker, he was a man of his word," and he "just carried so much moral authority." The co-op's board met twice a month to manage expenses, make purchases, and oversee policies. In order to be representative

[34] Hatch, "Historical Sketch and Progress Report on the North Bolivar County Farm Cooperative," *DHC*; Dorsey, "North Bolivar County Farm Cooperative, A. A. L., 1969 Progress Report," *DHC*; Black, *People and Plows*, 92–93; Interview with H. Jack Geiger by Robert Korstad and Neil Boothby; Interview with L. C. Dorsey by Robert Korstad and Neil Boothby.

[35] *People and Plows*, 93; Bill Rose, "Court Eyes Delta Food," *Delta-Democrat Times* (Greenville, Miss.), March 31, 1971, p. 1; Bill Rose, "Many Ways Tried to Salvage DFP," *Delta-Democrat Times* (Greenville, Miss.), March 31, 1971, p. 16.

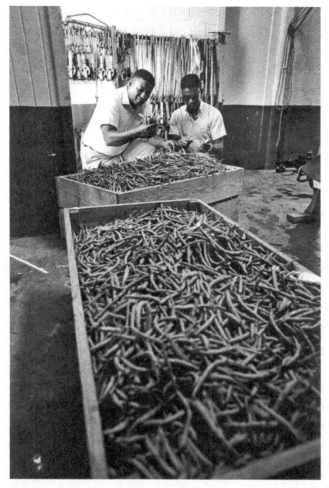

FIGURE 5.3 Co-op beans (Photo courtesy of Dan Bernstein, Southern Historical Collection, University of North Carolina at Chapel Hill).

of all the people it served—and to prevent the board from being dominated by traditional community leaders, such as ministers and school teachers—the board specifically recruited sharecroppers to join. The board recommended that each co-op club have at least one representative from each of the following categories:

1. A man older than seventy years of age and dependent on old-age assistance or Social Security
2. A woman older than seventy years of age and dependent on old-age assistance or Social Security
3. A female head of household with four or more school-age children in the home, and dependent on income within OEO's poverty guidelines

4. A male head of household under thirty years of age and dependent on income within poverty guidelines

5. A male head of household with four or more school-age children in the home and dependent on income within poverty guidelines

6. A housewife under thirty years of age dependent on income within poverty guidelines

7. A male between the ages of seventeen and twenty-one

8. A female between the ages of seventeen and twenty-one

9. Not more than five persons, without regard to income, might be chosen on the basis of known leadership qualities or whatever criteria the community felt appropriate for inclusion.[36]

Building membership across the county was one of the major goals and accomplishments of the board during its early years. One charter board member recalled going door-to-door throughout the county, explaining how the farm co-op worked and getting families to pay the one dollar membership fee. Surprisingly, even a small number of white members joined. John Hatch saw the co-op as an interesting entrée for breaking down some black–white barriers in the Delta: "Some poor whites . . . could deal with being in the field and working side by side with blacks because they'd done it in cotton and other things. It was kind of surprising to me that they would be more comfortable joining the cooperative than they would coming to the health center."[37]

In 1969 over 300 people worked for the co-op in one way or another, some earning cash or food for daily work on the farm, while others in both full- and part-time positions worked in all aspects of the co-op's operation. Along with jobs on the farm itself, the co-op provided a number of other opportunities for Bolivar County's poor. The frozen food locker employed a number of full-time workers, and others worked at the co-op stores established in Mound Bayou, Winstonville, Symonds, Rosedale, and Round Lake. "We set up co-op stores [where] the vegetables that we grew on the farm were delivered to and distributed to members in those communities," remembered L. C. Dorsey, "and a member was selected by the local community to run the store." These stores distributed the farm's produce to members and

[36] L. C. Dorsey Interview, Delta Health Center Tapes; *North Bolivar Farmers Coop* (n.p., n.d), *DHC*; North Bolivar County Farm Cooperative self-help nutritional program. Grant proposal (written by John Hatch), 1972, *JHP*; Mrs. Young Oral History; Ward interview with Hatch and Geiger; John Hatch interview with Rev. Ward.

[37] Mrs. Young Oral History; Interview with John Brown by John Hatch; Interview with John Hatch by Robert Korstad and Neil Boothby.

sold surplus to the public, while also reselling donated clothes. Winstonville was the first co-op store to offer recycled clothes to members; it hired one employee to work the store three days a week. Clothes were priced from five cents to two dollars an item, but the neediest buyers could receive clothes at no cost. Mrs. Lucinda Young, a charter member of the co-op board, recalled that, "A lot of people can't get through the winter, just like this lady got children and don't have clothes, we give her a referral to go to either one of those co-op stores and get clothes for herself or for her children." The clothes were donated from both around the state and around the nation, especially after the *LIFE* magazine article on the health center brought national attention to the plight of Bolivar County's poor. "Sometimes we have 80 or 100 boxes [of clothes] that come in," recalled Mrs. Young. "Plenty of them be new shoes."[38]

The co-op also operated a sandwich shop and a bookstore. The sandwich shop, located at the health center, drew a regular clientele of patients and employees every day, and it provided full-time employment for two co-op members. The African-American book and record store in Mound Bayou employed two full-time workers. All employees at the co-op stores were selected by their local co-op associations on the basis of need, in line with L. C. Dorsey's view of the co-op as an endeavor "that works hard on developing people, rather than working on a program. We try to take people, in the co-op, that might not get a job in other programs because of not enough formal education, a lot of other stupid stuff, and we put him into that program and they become involved and get an opportunity to develop without the fear of competition [with people of higher education]. . . ." As with the health center, the jobs created, with support from the federal government, injected needed cash into the local economy and helped break the cycle of poverty among poor blacks in the Delta.[39]

In the midst of its early successes, the Tufts–Delta Health Center and its farm co-op received national media attention. Some attention came about organically, but a fair share also stemmed from Jack Geiger's earlier career as a journalist. As Geiger wrote in a letter to Dr. Joe English, Director of Health Affairs at OEO in 1968, health centers "would need all the support and mass media coverage they could get in order to build the public base of knowledge and support in advance of any struggle that might arise for their survival." Geiger's media Rolodex helped

---

[38] Interview with L. C. Dorsey by Robert Korstad and Neil Boothby; North Bolivar County Farm Co-op Records (Box 1, Folder 1), Wisconsin Historical Society, Madison, Wisc.; *North Bolivar Farmers Coop* (n.p., n.d), *DHC*; Mrs. Young Oral History.

[39] North Bolivar County Farm Co-op Records, Wisconsin Historical Society; Interview with L. C. Dorsey by Robert Korstad and Neil Boothby; "The Delta Health Center Digest," *DHC*.

shine a bright light on the good works of the community health centers, with a special focus on Mound Bayou. As a result of his efforts, in late 1968 and 1969 there were articles on the Tufts–Delta Health Center in magazines and newspapers across the country, including *The Wall Street Journal, TIME, LOOK, LIFE, The New York Times, The Boston Globe*, and *The Washington Post*. Additionally, Associated Press coverage of the health center resulted in articles on the center reprinted in newspapers across the nation.[40]

This widespread media attention found an unlikely audience in the person of Monseigneur John Romaniello, a 69-year-old Catholic priest who had spent much of his career as a missionary in China. Expelled from mainland China as the communists took power, he moved to Hong Kong, where he tended to Chinese refugees with Catholic Relief Services. Part of his work in Hong Kong involved collaborating with local machinists to develop automated systems for turning flour (donated by the U.S. government) into noodles. Eventually, Romaniello set up seventeen "noodle stations" (each with its own large machine) throughout Hong Kong, which together produced as much as a million pounds of noodles per month for as many as 400,000 refugees.[41]

Romaniello came into contact with the North Bolivar County Co-op by way of Laurence L. Winthrop, former editor of *The Boston Globe*. Having done stories about both the co-op and the "Noodle Priest" (as Romaniello was known), Winthrop suggested that a similar program would be useful in Mississippi. Geiger and Hatch got in touch with Romaniello in late 1969 and explained the work of the co-op to him. Arrangements were made to send an old noodle machine to Mound Bayou, and in the summer of 1970, the machine, and later Fr. Romaniello, arrived in Mississippi.

The production of noodles in the Delta ran into a number of roadblocks. First, there was, at the time, no place to house the machine, which was much larger than anyone at the health center had envisioned. Secondly, Romaniello had planned on using U.S. government surplus flour, as he did in Hong Kong, but found that while the American government would provide him flour for noodles to feed hungry children in Hong Kong, it would not do so for hungry children in Mississippi. Frustrated, he left Mound Bayou, fearful that the Mississippi noodle project would never get off the ground.[42]

It took more than a year after Fr. Romaniello's first visit to Mississippi before noodles were produced for Bolivar County's poor, but eventually it did

[40] Letter from Geiger to Joseph English, November 19, 1968, *JGC*.

[41] Owen Taylor, "Mississippi, Meet the Noodle," *Delta Democrat-Times* (Greenville, Miss.), Nov. 11, 1971; "MSGR. JOHN ROMANIELLO," *New York Times*, October 25, 1985.

[42] Black, *People and Plows Against Hunger*, 55–57.

happen. Davis Taylor, then the publisher of *The Boston Globe*, established "Noodles for America," a charitable foundation dedicated to providing food to hungry Americans. With funding from Noodles for America and the OEO, the co-op was able to construct a building to house the noodle machine and purchase flour, and on November 10, 1971, noodle production began. The machine, which took two men to operate, could produce up to a ton of noodles a day. John Hatch hoped that the noodles, made from high protein soy, would help supplement the diets of Bolivar County's poor, especially in the winter months. He also understood the obstacle he faced in getting Delta residents to try a food that was very foreign to them: "Like spinach, that took almost three years for people to get used to, we do not expect members to immediately fall in love with noodles." Still, Hatch focused on the upside: "The only solution to malnutrition is food and a knowledge of how it can be prepared. This doesn't come automatically, but must be part of an elaborate teaching process . . . via people they know, instead of outside strangers. It goes into humble places that are familiar like churches, homes, [and] large halls."[43]

* * *

By 1970, the North Bolivar County Farm Co-op had 909 member families, the peak membership in its history. As the farm expanded its land holdings, it developed a double-planting method which allowed the co-op to provide members with fresh vegetables ten months out of the year: In the spring, the co-op planted peas, corn, cabbage, okra, lima beans, squash, cucumbers, and sweet potatoes; in the fall, cabbage, collards, turnips, peas, and lima beans. However, as the farm settled in agriculturally, it faced numerous pressures. Funding was the most difficult obstacle facing the farm in the early 1970s. When it was established, the North Bolivar County Co-op received start-up funding from the Office of Economic Opportunity with the understanding that it would eventually become a self-sustaining operation. OEO funding, however, was predicated on the co-op's ability to deliver various welfare-oriented benefits, but this requirement made achieving self-sufficiency more difficult. In addition to OEO funding, during its early years the co-op received donations from a wide variety of nongovernmental organizations, including the Ford Foundation and Measure for Measure, as well as corporations such as Green Giant and Coca-Cola. The co-op also received monetary support from private donors, including some local white plantation owners, many of whom donated anonymously. When federal support for the co-op—as with the health center and many other War on Poverty

[43] Black, *People and Plows*, 57–58; Taylor, "Mississippi, Meet the Noodle"; Hatch, "North Bolivar County Farm Cooperative Self-Help Nutritional Program," *DHC*.

projects throughout the nation—was dramatically reduced or eliminated under the Nixon administration, the co-op suffered. In 1972, all OEO grants to the co-op ended.[44]

Another limitation on the co-op's success was what L. C. Dorsey identified as the "plantation mentality" of many of the co-op members, who had a difficult time understanding that they were the owners of the co-op, not just employees; that the land was theirs, and what they produced was theirs. "Some people who come in and they still have the same types of hang-ups they had on the man's plantation," said Dorsey. "They see Mr. [John] Brown not as a member, [not] an equal member [of the co-op], but as the boss man. Or they will come and say things to me like, 'Here's the boss lady, what's she got to say?'" Many people had a difficult time grasping that the farm manager and the other paid employees of the co-op worked *for* them, and not the other way around. They "participated, gave free labor for vegetables, worked, brought in people, and never accepted that they were working for themselves," lamented Dorsey.[45]

This lack of understanding of how the co-op worked had practical ramifications, as the co-op struggled to get enough workers and efficiently deliver its vegetables to members. Initially, the co-op paid workers in both cash and credit that they could redeem for vegetables. By 1969, in order to attract and keep more workers, the co-op switched entirely to cash payments, without success. In their study of the co-op, Finney and McGranahan found that "the Cooperative had started out with a surplus of people willing to work. By 1970, however, . . . the Coop encountered increasing difficulties in mobilizing adequate numbers of workers when they were needed and in training them to pick according to standards of quality control." Vegetables rotted both in the field and at retail vegetable stands throughout north Bolivar County that operated a few days a week during the harvest season.[46]

In an attempt to save the operation co-op leaders turned away from the farm's original model of just having local people work the farm to produce food for themselves and their community and transitioned to the production of cash crops. Cash crops first were planted in 1969, when some of the co-op's land was used to plant cotton and soybeans, and continued to expand in the following years, while acreage to produce vegetables for distribution to co-op members gradually declined. The planting of cash crops demanded the use of heavy machinery, which, in turn, reduced the number of jobs available at the co-op, limiting positions to those who had certain machinery skills, such as driving a tractor or operating heavy farm equipment. These

---

[44] Finney and McGranahan, "Community Support and Goal Displacement in a Poor Peoples' Cooperative Farm," 20–21; John Hatch Notes, *JHC*.

[45] L. C. Dorsey Interview. Delta Health Center Tapes; Dorsey interview with Korstad and Boothby.

[46] Finney and McGranahan, "Community Support and Goal Displacement," 22–24.

changes moved the co-op dramatically away from its original mission of providing an outlet for the poor to work the land and get paid in either cash or food. Over the next few years, as the co-op increased its production of cash crops, the wages it paid out to day laborers declined dramatically, from $35,000 in 1969, to $25,000 in 1970 and 1971, and then $20,000 in 1972. Meanwhile, the wages paid to machine operators on the farm doubled.[47]

This change in focus resulted in criticism of the co-op's leadership as well as declining support among its members. From its peak membership of 909 families in 1970, membership in the co-op slid to only 500 families by the end of 1972. "They really tried to move away from supplying the needs of the poor people," recalled John Brown. Many of the welfare-orientated programs run by the co-op that had been popular with many members—including the African-American bookstore, resale clothing stores, meat locker, and the frozen food locker—were all closed by 1971, mainly because they were financial drags on the larger operation. "The co-op has been criticized as not being well-run, of being a plantation, and many other things," admitted L. C. Dorsey in 1971. "Maybe we're guilty of all these things, but we started out to fulfill a need that was expressed by our members."[48]

Having earned a high school equivalency certificate through the health center in 1968, L. C. Dorsey left Mound Bayou in 1971 to pursue a master's degree at the School of Social Welfare at SUNY-Stony Brook; after earning her MSW in 1973, she went on to earn her doctorate in social work from Howard University and complete further graduate work at Johns Hopkins University, where she earned a certificate in health care management. It was her experience at Stony Brook that allowed Dorsey to, in her words, "learn writing, grammar, and expression." [49]

John Brown was ousted in 1972 at the behest of OEO leadership following an audit of the co-op that recommended Brown be replaced by someone more experienced with farm management. Critics of Brown's leadership pointed out that although he had worked as a farm supervisor for eighteen years before coming to the co-op, he lacked experience making management decisions. Brown's removal caused deep divisions among the co-op board, who were torn between their friendship and loyalty to Brown and the financial pressure from OEO. He was succeeded as farm manager by Ronald Thornton, a Vietnam veteran who had studied agriculture and

[47] Finney and McGranahan, "Community Support and Goal Displacement," 15, 20–21; Black, *People and Plows*, 33–34, 70.

[48] Interview with John Brown, Southern Historical Collection; Finney and McGranahan, "Community Support and Goal Displacement," 21; L. C. Dorsey, "The North Bolivar County Health Cooperative," *Compared to What?: The TUFTS–Delta Health Center Newsletter*, DHC.

[49] "From Plantation to Law School: She Thinks This Trip is Necessary," *The New York Times* (Feb. 14, 1973); Karen Rutherford, "L. C. Dorsey," *The Mississippi Writers Page* (http://www.olemiss.edu/mwp/dir/dorsey_lc/).

business administration at Tuskegee University. Thornton was joined by another
Tuskegee graduate, Wendell Paris, who served as the new project director. Thornton
and Paris inherited a farm co-op with declining membership, the loss of federal
funding, and an operating deficit of over $18,000. They were greatly aided, however,
by news in the fall of 1972 that the co-op would receive a new $60,000 grant from
the federal government for a special nutrition project operated jointly by the co-op
and the health center. The money saved the co-op for the time being, and Paris and
Thornton worked hard to rebuild membership by returning the farm to more vegetable planting, but by the mid-1970s a string of wet seasons and more federal cuts
had placed the co-op in desperate straits. Beset by both massive funding cuts and
internal dissention about its direction, the co-op was never able to fulfill its promise
to be a self-sustaining operation, and it was eventually turned over to the historically
black Alcorn State University, which still manages it today as a research farm.[50]

Despite its ultimate failure to provide a long-term solution to feeding the poor
people of Bolivar County, the importance of the North Bolivar County Farm
Co-op in empowering the poor people of the Delta cannot be overstated; it was
simply the most creative and ambitious venture that sprung from the establishment
of the Tufts–Delta Health Center. "The pride of the people and being part of the
cooperative, part of something is all-black, and for blacks, and black-run is tremendous . . . [and] a lot people join[ed] just for that," recalled Dorsey. "There's a lot of
middle-class people that don't really need the benefits, don't fall into the criteria for
membership, but say, 'I just want to contribute; can I have an honorary membership? I think it is a wonderful black organization.'" Although separate from the
Tufts–Delta Health Center, the co-op was rooted in the optimism and creativity of
the health center's founders, especially John Hatch. As Dorsey later said of her one-
time nemesis, "John Hatch . . . is one of the few people I've met in life who is not
inhibited in dreaming. He doesn't care what anyone else thinks about his dreams
or his ideas or his notions. And he looked at this whole phenomenon of people on
some of the richest land in the country, perhaps even in the world, and couldn't
reconcile [them] starving to death. And he . . . [tried] to figure out what could be
done about it." Hatch's vision, and doggedness, helped former sharecroppers make
decisions about the land and crops, and allowed them to benefit directly from their
use. The farm co-op was, as historian John Dittmer wrote, "Where the traditional
public health center dispensed pills and shots, at Mound Bayou the staff attacked
the root causes of poor health and deprivation."[51]

---

[50] Brown, *People and Plows*, 35–37, 63–71.
[51] Dittmer, *The Good Doctors*, 233; L. C. Dorsey interview with Korstad and Boothby.

The Tufts–Delta Health Center fulfilled the goals of the Black Power movement more completely than the black–controlled health program that Mound Bayou's political leaders proposed. Yet the OEO was persuaded that blackness alone qualified people to run programs for African Americans and turned the project over to a group that did not adequately represent or serve the poor.

GRETA DEJONG[1]

6

Conflict and Change

DESPITE THE SUCCESSES of the Tufts–Delta Health Center, it remained a controversial program in Mississippi and faced opposition to its very existence from a variety of quarters, some expected and some not. By the early 1970s, the local opposition to the health center aligned with the national political climate, in which all Great Society programs were under assault following the election of President Richard Nixon. As a result of these changes, the health center's founding institutions and individuals, including Jack Geiger and Tufts University, eventually removed themselves from the business of healthcare delivery in north Bolivar County.

Opposition from Mississippi politicians and most white physicians was a relative constant from the inception of the health center, and this opposition continued even after the center was built and services were being delivered to the Delta poor. Mississippi's governor initially had refused to approve the center's application as a nonprofit corporation, forcing Tufts to establish the center as a charitable trust (which did not need the governor's signature). In addition, there were repeated attempts by Mississippi's congressional delegation to have the center's funding cut or eliminated. In September of 1968, Dr. R. T. Hollingsworth of Shelby wrote Mississippi's U.S. Senator John Stennis, thanking him "for all the help you gave us a couple of years ago in trying to prevent the Tufts Medical Project from being

---

[1] DeJong, "Plantation Politics," 275.

established at Mound Bayou." However, he continued, as "all of our best efforts failed and the Tufts Delta Medical Center is now a reality . . . I would like to beg you to use your influence to have the appropriate government agencies take a long hard look into the governments [*sic*] operations in the medical field in the Mound Bayou area." Stennis, who deemed the Tufts–Delta Health Center "an obvious waste of money," promised Hollingsworth that he would "use all of my influence on the Appropriations Committee to see that this project gets a thorough going over. Nevertheless, now that these people have their foot in the door, it might be difficult to slam it shut."[2]

Obstruction from state officials continued throughout Tufts–Delta Health Center's existence, including surveillance of the center and its staff by the State Sovereignty Commission. Much of this opposition was part of a general defiance to the War on Poverty by Mississippi politicians, but much of the hostility was specific to the health center and the belief that it was little more than a cover for civil rights activities. Sen. Stennis, an erstwhile opponent of all Great Society programs in Mississippi, ordered a number of investigations into the health center's finances over the years, including investigations that center staff and vehicles were used to help support black political campaigns.[3] The advent of Medicare and Medicaid—programs vehemently opposed by Mississippi's Congressional delegation—also increased opposition from some white physicians in the Mississippi Delta toward the health center, because some now sought—most for the first time—to recruit black patients to their practices, now that the federal government was paying for their health insurance.

While resistance from Mississippi politicians and white physicians had been expected, the most unexpected criticisms and interference came from the black community of Bolivar County. The health center was a contentious topic for locals, shining a light on and even exacerbating class divisions among blacks that negatively impacted the center for years. John Hatch once openly questioned "whether poor blacks and middle-class blacks were significantly closer together" following the experience of the civil rights movement in Mississippi; he concluded that "they were not." Some of these conflicts rested on long-simmering class divisions between Mound Bayou's black elites and those who worked on the plantations, but most tensions surrounded the influx of federal money into the benighted region, and who

---

[2] Letter from R. T. Hollingsworth, MD, Shelby Community Hospital, Sept. 16, 1968, to Sen. Stennis; Letter from Sen. Stennis to R. T. Hollingsworth, MD, Shelby Community Hospital, Oct. 16, 1968. Both letters located in the John C. Stennis Collection, Special Collections, Mitchell Library, Mississippi State University, Series 25, Box 7, Folder 25.

[3] DeJong, "Plantation Politics," 267.

would get to control it. Author Greta DeJong found that "Mound Bayou's black leaders recognized the threats to their dominance posed by the economic and political empowerment of poor people and joined their white counterparts in efforts to undermine the project."[4]

One of the most influential figures in Mound Bayou at the time of the health center's opening was Earl Lucas, a Dillard University graduate who had returned home to try to develop new economic opportunities for blacks in the Delta. Lucas was then managing another OEO-funded initiative, Systematic Training and Redevelopment (STAR), an adult education and job placement program sponsored by the Catholic Church in Mississippi. "[Geiger] stopped at my house and talked with me at length about [the health center]," Lucas later recalled. "Initially, I was trying to help them to come to Mississippi and especially to Mound Bayou. . . . I was instrumental in getting the city government to annex some property for their protection, because most of the whites in the area thought it was socialized medicine." [5]

Although Geiger's relationship with Lucas seemed to start off on a good footing, it would soon sour, and Lucas would prove to be a tremendous thorn in the side of Geiger and the entire endeavor. Their first conflict centered on employment at the center. "[Lucas] was modestly enthusiastic about us in the beginning," remembered Geiger, "but then kept writing us and saying he wanted a specific list of our job openings, [even] as we were beginning to hire staff at every level and do all of this training." Lucas wanted Geiger to have STAR manage all the hiring for the health center. Geiger told him that such a proposal was unworkable, because the center had to be able to control its own hiring. "Our position," said Geiger, "was that . . . everybody was free to apply, but that we were not going to short circuit people from STAR that Earl would send. And that was the first kind of rift."[6]

Lucas's wife, Mary, a nurse, was an early hire at the Tufts–Delta Health Center. "[Registered nurses] were hard to come by, and a local one seemed to be a plus," recalled Geiger. "What we didn't know, of course, is that she regarded Tufts as an outside intruder on her own belief in her status as part of Mound Bayou's ruling elite." What Geiger and others at the health center soon came to realize was that, as part of the black upper class in Mound Bayou that had traditionally controlled most of the political and economic power in the black community, Earl and Mary Lucas viewed the health center as a great opportunity if they could control it—but a threat to their way of life if they could not. The black elites of Mound Bayou—elected

[4] Patton, "Community Health Centers: The Early Years of the Movement"; DeJong, "Plantation Politics," 268.
[5] Interview with Mayor Earl Lewis, Southern Historical Collection, UNC–Chapel Hill; Rodgers, *Life and Death in the Delta*, 152–53.
[6] Ward interview with Geiger; Sobelson, "Participation, Power, and Place," 81.

officials, teachers, and store owners—were a "caste within a caste system," said Dr. Bob Smith, and they "understood the dynamics of what political power and money meant in a society." Another tension, described by L. C. Dorsey, was that while many of people associated with the Tufts–Delta Health Center—including herself, Jack Geiger, and Bob Smith—had been "movement people," activists on the front lines during the civil rights campaigns of the early 1960s, most of the middle-class blacks who traditionally controlled jobs in Mound Bayou "were the same people who had refused to join the demonstrations in the early, dangerous days."[7]

In her study of the health center, DeJong wrote that, "The economic and political interests of Mound Bayou's black middle class were threatened by antipoverty projects and the political mobilization they generated." Some of this tension revolved around status, but more of it centered on money. In fact, many of President Johnson's fears regarding the OEO's Community Action programs, especially those related to award-ing public money to private agencies, proved to be true in Bolivar County. The control of the health center, and the federal dollars that it brought in, was a major source of friction, but the economic impact on the community was also unsettling to many in the traditional leadership class. Jack Cartwright, who worked at the center, summa-rized this problem: "You got 15 people off this plantation working at the center, quite naturally Mr. John Doe's going to get upset because he's losing some of his labor."[8]

The pay employees at the health center received was an even more significant issue than the loss of farm labor in the Delta. By federal law, the health center had to pay its employees at least minimum wage, which represented a dramatic increase for most Delta blacks. One local white attorney, an informant for the State Sovereignty Commission, reported that the health center had created "untold dissention among the citizenry of and around Mound Bayou" by paying people salaries that were far above prevailing labor rates.[9]

Black women employed at the Tufts–Delta Health Center, who prior to its founding had few options other than domestic work at near starvation wages (and who were often subject to sexual exploitation by their male employers, black or white), now earned a wage comparable to local school teachers. "From 15 dollars a week to 300-and-some dollars every two weeks, to me that was a blessing," re-called Barbara Brooks, an early employee of the center. Such changes caused resent-ment among some local black elites who previously had held economic, political, and social sway over their impoverished neighbors. Geiger recounted an incident in

[7] Sobelson, "Participation, Power, and Place," 76, 81; Dorsey, *Freedom Came to Mississippi*, 33.

[8] DeJong, "Plantation Politics," 256–57; Stossel, *Sarge*, 375–76; Interview with Barbara Brooks and Jack Cartwright.

[9] DeJong, "Plantation Politics," 267–68.

which a gun-toting local man, obviously intoxicated, stormed into the health center demanding to see "Mr. Tufts," who had "stolen his woman." The woman in question had been his maid who had quit her job and escaped the sexual exploitation that came with it when she was hired at the health center. She "could now tell him . . . [that] he could take that job and shove it," recalled Geiger.[10]

The opposition of many in the black middle class to the improved station of the black poor was something that most organizers of the health center had not antici-pated. "They resented the fact that we were putting in screen doors and windows and patching up houses for people who lived on plantations," stated L. C. Dorsey. "They resented the fact that we had taken women who were working for them for 12 and 15 dollars a week and had given them jobs." Dorsey continued, "It was a resent-ment that I don't think that those of us from outside of Mound Bayou fully appreci-ated and understood. I mean, we had no prior experiences to prepare us for this kind of classism, this kind of isolation . . . and we just weren't prepared for that."[11]

Certainly not all members of Mound Bayou's leadership class were opposed to either the Tufts–Delta Health Center or improving conditions for the local black poor. "There were established Mound Bayou people very much in support of us," Geiger recalled. But many local leaders, black and white, sought to frustrate the efforts of the health center, the health associations, and the co-op. Pressure was ap-plied to locals by those John Hatch classified as "gatekeeper blacks"— ministers, school teachers, and business owners—who had reservations about disrupting the local status quo. Hatch recounted a humorous incident in which a local preacher, who cautiously had been allowing his church to be used as a meeting place for the Round Lake Health Association, changed his mind. "The preacher got antsy—*all these meetings, what are they talking about? Freedom and voting and stuff?*" recalled Hatch. "And, you know, white folk were putting a few dollars in his pocket. So he decided Miss Pearl and Mr. Sam [were] no longer assets. So he put a padlock on the church door." Miss Pearlia B. Robinson, who was a member of the church, did not take well to the situation, and, in turn, put another padlock on the church door, locking the minister out of his own church. "This eventually led to an unlocking ceremony and peacemaking," recalled Hatch with a laugh, and the health associa-tion meetings resumed shortly thereafter.[12]

Not all conflicts were solved so amicably, and tensions between the health center and local officials escalated as the center gained influence in the area. By 1970 the

---

[10] Interview with Barbara Brooks and Jack Cartwright; Interview with H. Jack Geiger by Robert Korstad and Neil Boothby; Sobelson, "Participation, Power, and Place," 76–77.

[11] Interview with L. C. Dorsey by Robert Korstad and Neil Boothby.

[12] Sobleson, "Participation, Power, and Place," 80; Ward interview with Geiger and Hatch.

relationship between Earl Lucas, by then mayor of Mound Bayou, and the Tufts–Delta Health Center became so toxic that the city tried to appropriate taxes from the tax-exempt facility, even threatening to build a sewage lagoon next to the health center. Lucas denied that he sought to tax the health center, but instead insisted that "most institutions like this give services to the community in lieu of taxes. That's what we wanted." Lucas had requested that the health center provide a "Community Assistance Program" to the town in lieu of taxes, including an economic assistance package and an environmental services package, as well as the donation of a garbage truck and a fire truck to the town. In response, Andrew James, at this time the director of the health center, asserted that, "We have to consider the other towns that we serve as well as Mound Bayou," and detailed numerous examples of services that he and his staff at the center had provided the town for years, including regular inspections of Mound Bayou's water and sewage systems, and the matter was eventually dropped. The city government's threat to put its sewage lagoon next to the health center's property was more troubling. After some tense negotiations, James reported that, "Our environmental health service and two engineers from Tufts University . . . [eventually] worked with the town and its engineers to revise the plan."[13]

Tied to the tensions over federal money and control of the health center was the Mound Bayou Community Hospital, created out of the merger of the two old fraternal hospitals and funded by an OEO grant separate from that of the Tufts–Delta Health Center. Geiger did not ever intend for the health center to compete with the Mound Bayou Community Hospital, but rather to complement it. "Hospitals usually can't and don't do what health centers do; they can't do home care, home nursing, outreach programs over 500 square mi. area, community organization, health counsel formation," wrote Geiger. "On the other hand, health centers can't do in-hospital care, the intensive care of acute and chronic illness, surgery and all the other functions hospitals provide; and every health center program should be connected with the hospital for these purposes. The one place in Mississippi where a health center–hospital relationship was possible was Mound Bayou."[14] Not everyone agreed with Geiger's assessment of the relationship between the two institutions. Those who wanted to see the health center closed down, like the governor of Mississippi, and those who wanted to see it—and its federal funding—subsumed by the Mound Bayou Community Hospital, including many of those who had run the old fraternal hospitals, argued that the hospital and the health center provided

---

[13] Laura Cefalu, "Tufts Center, Mound Bayou hospital clash," *Delta Democrat-Times*, October 19, 1970; Letter from Earl Lucas to Andrew James, August 4, 1970, *JGC*.

[14] Letter to Samuel Nixon, Meharry medical student, from Jack Geiger, n.d., Series 1, Subseries 1, Box 8, Folder 60, *DHC*.

an unnecessary, and fiscally unsound, duplication of services. It would be better, the opponents of the health center argued, for the federal money to go just to the hospital, and its board, rather than having the services, and the money, divided between the two institutions.

This struggle between the hospital and the health center over issues of money, control, and competence was a constant source of strife. One of the earliest struggles developed between the physicians at the Tufts–Delta Health Center, most of whom were young and had been well-trained at some of the nation's best medical schools and hospitals, and those at the Mound Bayou Community Hospital, who were older and had been subjected to tremendous professional isolation from practicing in the Jim Crow South. It is important to remember that not all of Mississippi's black physicians had been activists like Bob Smith and Aaron Shirley; in fact, throughout the Jim Crow South, most black physicians had steered clear of civil rights activities and pursued a markedly conservative attitude toward the movement. Their inaction is not entirely surprising—they had overcome seemingly insurmountable odds to make a career in the segregated South, and the changes brought on by the civil rights movement, especially the end of segregated facilities such as all-black hospitals, threatened both their status and livelihoods.

Nowhere was this situation more apparent than with the physicians who ran the Taborian and Sara Brown Hospitals. For decades they had provided the Delta's black population with a modicum of care, which, while certainly inadequate in many respects, was vital and a source of pride to the local black community. For these physicians, who had been denied staff and admitting privileges at public hospitals throughout their careers, small, black-owned and run hospitals like Taborian and Sara Brown were central to their professional and economic survival, and these hospitals had allowed them to carve out both personal and professional status within their community. It is no wonder that the arrival of younger, better-trained physicians, backed by federal dollars, presented a threat to them, and they reacted defensively.

Geiger understood, rightfully, that the arrival of the health center posed an economic threat to the town's local physicians, Drs. Burton and Lowery. Bob Smith explained that black physicians in Mississippi—including himself—were making $5,000 a year or less in the mid-1960s. When the Tufts project came in, its physicians—who were paid by the federal government and had appointments as Tufts Medical School faculty—were making more than $30,000 a year. "It created a hell of a lot of tensions in the sense that, on one hand, the motives [of Tufts] were right, but the reality was that we had two black physicians there who were the head of these hospitals, who were making nothing," recalled Smith. "It was more of what black people saw as typifying America."[15]

[15] Sobelson, "Participation, Power, and Place," 77–78.

Geiger sought to mitigate this problem by offering the two doctors the possibility of a quarter-time association with the health center. In November 1967, while the health center was still operating out of the church parsonage, Dr. Burton called Geiger and asked for his check—asserting that he had been promised a retainer as a "payoff." Geiger (and later Meharry's Matthew Walker) told Drs. Burton and Lowery that such a payoff would be both immoral and illegal, and that the center would not pay anyone for services not rendered. Geiger did, however, ask the OEO to provide both of the local physicians $2,000 a year for their care of health center patients who were admitted to the community hospital. This stipend was approved by OEO and helped smooth the situation over, but it was emblematic of some of the strains between the center and the hospital.[16]

On the other hand, many of the younger physicians, both black and white, but especially white non-Southerners who had been trained in modern facilities outside the South, found the condition of the facilities—including broken windows permitting flies into the operating room and a lack of modern equipment—appalling. Furthermore, they complained about the inadequate staff training and the practices of the local physicians, and were often unable to hide their displeasure with either. Even the Meharry residents who rotated through Mound Bayou for three-month periods understood the inadequacies of the hospital. One told a reporter from *The Boston Globe*, "If it is a routine case and there are no complications we are alright. If it is a complex case, or something goes sour—then we are in over our head because we lack equipment and staff."[17]

Although rightfully critical of the fiefdoms that some of these physicians had built, the lack of understanding of what these older black physicians and black hospitals had done for their community over the long and difficult period that preceded the civil rights era contributed to the tensions between the two groups. Geiger exacerbated these tensions when, in a 1969 interview with *LIFE* magazine, he stated that "I guess we were practicing missionary medicine. . . . We work at creating a comprehensive health program where virtually none existed. Our aim was to use health as a basis, a point of entry into the poverty cycle that would eventually lead to broader social change."[18] The comment did not go over well with those at Meharry or the Mound Bayou Community Hospital, which had both been delivering medical care to the region for decades. In a letter to the editor of *LIFE*, a Meharry student named Samuel C. Nixon II responded, " 'A stir of hope'—not until Tufts?

---

[16] Sobelson, "Participation, Power, and Place," 77–78; Letter to Anne Haendel, OEO, from Geiger (October 9, 1968), Series 1, Subseries 1, Box 1, Folder 2, *DHC*.

[17] "New Hospital is First Tangible By-Product of Tufts Project," *Boston Globe*, July 18, 1967.

[18] Hall, "A Stir of Hope in Mound Bayou," 73.

Ridiculous! Meharry Medical College, a small, black, poor but excellent medical school, has sent externs, interns and residents to Mound Bayou for more than a decade, long before 'wealthy' Tufts University and OEO dreamed of going there."[19]

Geiger had to backtrack his statements with both Meharry's leadership and the physicians and residents at the hospital; he also wrote a personal letter to Samuel Nixon. He explained that he was referring to the work that the Tufts–Delta Health Center was doing for uninsured patients in the rural areas—those who had been too poor to even be able to afford the hospital insurance provided by the fraternal orders and often had been turned away at Taborian and Sara Brown. In many ways, however, the damage was done.

In order to try to mend the relationship with Meharry, Geiger helped write an OEO grant for what became the Matthew Walker Community Health Center in Nashville. As part of the grant, a new department of community medicine also was established at Meharry. "I think that repaired the breach to some extent," Geiger later recalled, but his comment soured relations among the center, the hospital, and Meharry for years to come, even after Geiger had left Mound Bayou.[20]

This combination of fear and resentment from local black physicians and hospital administrators toward the Tufts staff, along with the dissatisfaction that many at the health center had toward those at the Mound Bayou Community Hospital, created a volatile situation. Adding to this tension was the large amount of federal money that was being poured into Mound Bayou with the arrival of Tufts. "When Tufts got involved in Mound Bayou it just seemed like truckloads of money were available," and the perception that "outsiders" controlled most of it left a "bitter taste in the mouths of Meharry" and others in the town, according to L. C. Dorsey.[21] The large amount of federal funding spent on the Tufts–Delta Health Center—controlled by a "white" institution from Massachusetts, new to the Mississippi Delta—caused resentment from the black-run institutions that had been providing medical care in Mound Bayou for decades. Real or not, there was also resentment of a perceived paternalistic attitude by the Tufts leadership toward the leaders of Mound Bayou, the community hospital, and Meharry, which contributed to the often icy relationship. Criticism of the hospital care, and the "missionary medicine" comment in *LIFE*, added to the tension, despite the civil rights *bona fides* of Geiger and other members of the Tufts staff.

The tensions between the old guard and the Tufts–Delta Health Center had negative impacts on the care that each institution was able to provide. The Mound

---

[19] "Letters to the Editor," *LIFE* (April 18, 1969), 22B.
[20] Interview with H. Jack Geiger by Tom Ward.
[21] Sobelson, "Participation, Power, and Place," 79–80.

Bayou Community Hospital continued to operate under the old fraternal hospital system—selling its insurance and charging nonmembers for service, even though its OEO grant mandated that poverty patients had to be cared for at no charge. (Indeed, their adherence to the old way was signaled by the fact that the large "Taborian Hospital" sign above the entrance was never removed.) Geiger protested that, "Black people who were in poverty—but not fraternal order members—[were] often turned away at the admitting office, or [told that a] $50 cash advance was required." As a result, he recalled, "Although fraternal members were only a small part of the population, they remain[ed] the majority of the hospital patients." Sister Mary Stella echoed Geiger's complaints, writing that "[The hospital] just sent us a letter saying that they could not take any more unwed mothers. Why? They don't want to 'get a bad name for themselves.'" Those who were referred to the hospital from the health center often complained that the hospital's doctors and staff mistreated them, labeling them "Tufts patients" and asking them to pay for services that were supposed to be free.[22]

Eventually, William Maloney, Dean of the Tufts Medical School, codified the collected frustrations with the community hospital and its fraternal network in a letter to an OEO official. He complained that because members of the fraternal orders were sitting in influential positions on the community hospital's board of directors, "the fraternal orders [are] effectively competing with the purposes of the O.E.O. grant by attempting to sell hospitalization insurance to the same population that is eligible either for totally free or partially-paid care at the hospital under the poverty program." In essence, Maloney contended, the fraternal leaders saw the OEO grant as little more than a bailout to allow them to continue business as usual; the Knights and Daughters of Tabor even distributed a flier proclaiming "Taborian Hospital Now Backed by Federal Government." Eventually, the OEO demanded the hospital board to print and distribute a brochure informing the poverty population specifically that free hospitalization was available under the OEO grant.[23]

This ongoing quality of care problem was also a persistent source of tension. Geiger wrote to OEO about a number of problems concerning care at the hospital, especially the oversight provided by the hospital's chief of surgery, Dr. Burton. In January of 1969, Geiger told the OEO's Anne Haendel that there had been a host of incidents at the hospital, including some that had resulted in the deaths of patients, which Geiger attributed to the incompetence of Dr. Burton and his staff.

[22] Letter to Samuel Nixon, Meharry medical student, from Jack Geiger, n.d. (1969?), Series 1, Subseries 1, Box 8, Folder 60, Delta Health Center Papers; Simpson, *Sister Stella's Babies*, 76; DeJong, "Plantation Politics," 270.
[23] Letter from William F. Maloney to Dr. Thomas Bryant, Assistant Director for Health Affairs, OEO, August 13, 1970, *JGC*.

Geiger also recounted incidents of operating rooms not being adequately staffed or equipped, writing, "We continue to find the hospital without the low elementary performance with regard to drug administration, temperature, weights, IV fluids and . . . other things." Finally, he complained that some members of the hospital staff actually ignored patients who had come to the hospital from the health center, stating, "They're a Tufts patient. We don't do anything for them." He concluded by telling Haendel: "We cannot continue much longer in good conscience to put patients and hospital under such circumstances."[24]

Geiger's criticisms of the hospital's care also caused friction between the health center and Meharry. The relationship between Meharry and Tufts was one that Geiger initially embraced as being a positive for the health center; he knew that without the aid of the Meharry residents, the Mound Bayou Community Hospital would not be able to handle the patient load that he expected it to receive. There were, however, long-standing tensions in Mississippi, Nashville, and Washington regarding the decision to have Tufts develop a health center—and receive millions in federal aid—when Meharry, a black institution, had been in Mound Bayou for over twenty years. Geiger had not criticized the Meharry residents in his letter to OEO—although he did note that they were routinely unsupervised—but the letter resulted in a response from Meharry's president, Dr. Lloyd C. Elam, who voiced his concern as to what was going on at the hospital, and even questioned whether he wanted the Meharry residents to continue serving in Mound Bayou. Geiger recommended to President Elam that the health center's physicians assume the role of attending physicians at the hospital, conduct daily morning rounds with the residents, and be on call for any problems. He couched his recommendation, however, telling Elam, "I hope [this proposal is] not perceived as crowding our way in or being condescending." Unfortunately, the school's dean, Dr. Ralph Cazort, did take offense to the letter, forcing Geiger to write Cazort an apology, stating "the intent of my earlier correspondence was never to be critical of the Meharry students, the surgical service at Mound Bayou Community Hospital, or Meharry itself; its sole purpose was to underscore the difficult problems at MBCH and to stress the need for additional professional input." The situation eventually died down, but the tensions between Meharry and the Tufts–Delta Health Center continued.[25]

---

[24] Letter to Anne Haendel, OEO, from Geiger (January 17, 1969), Series 1, Subseries 1, Box 8, Folder 58, *DHC*.

[25] Letter from Dr. Lloyd C. Elam, President, Meharry, to Geiger, February 3, 1969, Series 1, Subseries 1, Box 8, Folder 58, *DHC*; Letter from Geiger to Dr. Lloyd Elam, President of Meharry, Jan 27, 1969, Series 1, Subseries 1, Box 8, Folder 58, *DHC*; Letter from Geiger to Dr. Ralph Cazort, Dean, Meharry, Feb. 11, 1969, Series 1, Subseries 1, Box 8, Folder 58, *DHC*.

The health center, and especially Geiger, were also regularly criticized in the Mound Bayou *Voice*, the town's only paper. Geiger and his professional staff—most of whom were black—had to defend themselves repeatedly from attacks by members of the Mound Bayou city government and leaders of the Mound Bayou Community Hospital to OEO that their criticism of the hospital was racist and that they were exploiting the black poor of the Delta. Geiger was often derided in the Mound Bayou *Voice* as "a Tarzan" or "the boss man," who was duping the poor blacks who supported him and the health center. The constant conflicts with local authorities took its toll on Geiger and the other senior staff members, and Geiger confessed that he sometimes felt "consumed by the struggle" with local leaders.[26]

Although much of the conflict over the health center dealt with money and control of the facilities, race certainly played a role as well, even though the majority of the health center's staff, and much of its leadership, was black. The fact that a "white" university like Tufts—instead of a black institution like Meharry or the Mound Bayou town government—was in control of the center and its federal funding, and that a white physician was the face of the center, kept race at the forefront of many issues surrounding the Tufts–Delta Health Center. "People not knowing how the health center started," recalled Bob Smith, "started fighting the health center because there was people who felt that . . . 'Well, Meharry has been here for 20 years, 30 years, why don't you give the money to Meharry?'" In 1968, Dr. Mildred Morehead of Albert Einstein College of Medicine visited Mound Bayou to do an external, independent quality evaluation of both the Tufts–Delta Health Center and the Mound Bayou Community Hospital as part of a series of evaluations being done nationwide for OEO. Although her report described the health center as "superb" and the hospital as "abysmal," she concluded her report by recommending that all OEO monies for health care should be directed to the "black" hospital, and not the health center, which she said was run by "white outsiders." Geiger bitterly noted that her recommendations showed no regard for what was in the best interest of the poor, black patients of north Bolivar County.[27]

The issue of "white control" remained at the center of conflict over the health center and the hospital as OEO began to consider merging the two entities. Mound Bayou Mayor Earl Lucas repeatedly contacted OEO to assert that he and his colleagues were the only true representatives of the target population, and, because both of the facilities were in Mound Bayou, they should be run by the Mound Bayou city government, not by Tufts. Tensions culminated in August of 1968, when

---

[26] Sobelson, "Participation, Power, and Place," 80.

[27] H. Jack Geiger, "Chronology of Conflict in Mound Bayou," *JGC*; Ward interview with Dr. Robert Smith.

a delegation consisting of the hospital's board, Mayor Lucas, and other city officials went to Washington to meet with OEO officials to demand a merger of the hospital and the health center, with the merged facility being placed under their control. Dr. Sydney Maurer, who was serving as the acting director of OEO Health Affairs while Director Joe English was in Alaska, called Geiger to get his input. Geiger, who knew nothing of this meeting, immediately flew to Washington and told Maurer that any such change could only be approved by OEO and Tufts University, which was the current recipient of the grant. "I met with some of [the OEO people] afterward and said, 'You are destroying us, and you need to understand something about who these people are,'" remembered Geiger. "Well, at least they are black and from Mound Bayou," they told him.[28]

Geiger replied by pointing out that the Health Center Director, the Chief of Obstetrics and Gynecology, the Chief of Surgery, and two other staff physicians were black, as were the Directors of Nursing, Social Work, Pharmacy, Community Organizing and Health Education, Environmental Health Services, the laboratory, and the farm co-op. Furthermore, he maintained that 90 percent of the health center's staff consisted of black residents of Bolivar County, not just Mound Bayou, and, more importantly, that of the over 8,000 patients whom the center had seen since its inception, over 7,000 were not from Mound Bayou, but from the rest of north Bolivar County, and were, therefore, not represented by the Mound Bayou town government. Geiger further stressed that the focus should be on who was aiding and empowering the poor in Bolivar County. Under Tufts's leadership, he argued, the poor of Bolivar County, for the first time ever, had gained a seat at the table in the decisions being made about their health care, and the Tufts–Delta Health Center was, indeed, fulfilling the OEO mandate of "maximum feasible participation of the poor." Geiger lamented that much of the OEO leadership seemed to have no conception that the health center served a much larger area than Mound Bayou, or understand what the health center did for rural Bolivar County. Maurer then told them all to return to Mississippi and ordered the health center and hospital boards to come up with a plan for a merger.[29]

When OEO Health Director Joe English returned to Washington, Geiger set up a meeting between himself, English, and Dean William Maloney of Tufts Medical School. Geiger and Maloney asserted that to order a merger and change the authority of the Tufts–Delta Health Center from the existing grantee, Tufts, before the

---

[28] H. Jack Geiger, "Chronology of Conflict in Mound Bayou," *JGC*; Interview with Geiger by Korstad and Boothby.

[29] H. Jack Geiger, "Chronology of Conflict in Mound Bayou," *JGC*; Interview with Geiger by Korstad and Boothby.

grant was completed would be both unwise and illegal. English agreed, and rescinded Maurer's order. Upon hearing of the reversal, Mayor Lucas and Walter Wilson of the Knights and Daughters of Tabor flew to Washington to protest the reversal, but to no avail. English did, however, urge that the two facilities work together.[30]

In late 1968 and early 1969, in accordance with a mandate from the OEO for "cooperation and coordination" between the hospital and the health center, and in an attempt to improve patient care at the hospital, the clinicians of the Tufts–Delta Health Center formed a series of subcommittees with two Meharry residents and the staff at the Mound Bayou Community Hospital. Despite attempts at collaboration, however, a host of conflicts emerged between the two staffs, and in October 1969 all nine of the health center's clinicians sent a letter to OEO Project Analyst Anne Haendel describing numerous cases of gross quality errors that resulted in injuries, and even death, at the hospital. They argued that "cooperation and coordination" were inadequate to bring about real change, because neither Tufts nor Meharry had any effective means of improving the quality of care at the hospital. Instead, they asserted, it was the responsibility of the OEO, as the granting agency, to enforce quality standards on the hospital, its grantee.[31]

Cooperation and coordination continued to sour as tensions over control and OEO funding continued. In August of 1970 the conflict between the hospital and the health center reached its peak when Tufts Medical School Dean William Maloney ordered the health center's staff to cease the hospitalization of any of their patients at the Mound Bayou Community Hospital. In a letter to Dr. Thomas Bryant, the new Director of Health Affairs at OEO, Maloney referenced the October 1969 report wherein health center clinicians had documented quality-of-care issues at the hospital, including unnecessary injury and death to patients, and complained that "Eight months later, the situation remains essentially unchanged—and just as bad. . . . We are, increasingly, in the dangerous position of continuing to participate in an intolerable quality of care and being complicit in silence about it." Maloney also was scathingly critical of the OEO's handling of the hospital, asserting that "The past responses of O.E.O. to all of these problems, have, to us, been painful." He referenced a hospital site visit by the OEO in the wake of health center staff complaints, which found the quality of care "satisfactory," but he asserted that the OEO officials did not even ask the names of the patients who had complaints or pull their medical records.[32]

---

[30] H. Jack Geiger, "Chronology of Conflict in Mound Bayou," *JGC*.

[31] Ibid.

[32] Ibid.; Laura Cefalu, "Tufts Center, Mound Bayou hospital clash," *Delta Democrat-Times*, October 19, 1970.

"It is our judgment," wrote Maloney, "that quality of care will be impossible to accomplish with a board that sees the hospital as an economic enterprise . . . that is oriented almost entirely toward Mound Bayou itself—and the fraternal orders—rather than any larger or poorer population." He concluded with an ardent defense of Tufts's involvement in Mound Bayou, in light of the many racially oriented allegations that had been levied against it:

> We have often felt that O.E.O. was responding to the view that these were problems of an 'outside' 'white' institution being rejected by a black population that it served, or that O.E.O. was responding to charges that it was unfairly discriminating against a black institution, the hospital, and therefore trying to treat the two institutions as identical in both strengths and functions. In our opinion, the view that an outside white institution was being rejected is simply not true. We believe . . . that such attacks are an effort by a small, economically motivated and totally unrepresentative group in one community. Our own involvement with, and support from, the great bulk of the black population from northern Bolivar County is a matter of record.

The letter from Maloney to Bryant was leaked to, and then reprinted in, the Mound Bayou *Voice*, the local paper that long had been critical of the Tufts–Delta Health Center and its professional staff. The accompanying commentary that "this letter . . . might cause the community to loose [*sic*] all chances of getting the 150 bed hospital that it so desperately needs," further exacerbated the situation.[33]

Mayor Lucas responded to "The Letter," as it came to be known, by writing Dean Maloney demanding explanations for his accusations, even threatening a libel suit. The Letter also caused a great deal of consternation within the Tufts–Delta Health Center itself, as its message and tone divided staff and damaged morale. Dr. David Weeks, deputy director of the health center, wrote a confidential memo to Andrew James regarding the letter and its impact. He lamented that "key staff . . . were upset that they were not consulted in its timing or content and that its tone was overly strong." He worried that the letter's tone "projects an image of 'whitey telling blacks how to run their boards,'" which would only make matters worse between the hospital and the health center. Similar sentiments were expressed from the North Bolivar County Health Council, which asserted that the letter made it seem as policy was being set by "Tufts-Boston," and not the people of Bolivar County.[34]

---

[33] Cefalu, "Tufts Center, Mound Bayou hospital clash," *The Voice* [Mound Bayou, Miss.], October 6–20, 1970.

[34] Memo from David Weeks to Andrew James, September 1, 1970, *JGC*; Memo from Dave Caldwell and Ted Parish to William Crockett, September 18, 1970, *JGC*.

James, now the health center director, tried in earnest to smooth things over, couching the disagreements as personal rather than institutional. "Mat King [the hospital's administrator] and I aren't going to fight. Our commitments are to the communities and the people in this area. Tufts may leave the health center because of resources, but the center itself is permanent." Tufts's Maloney, too, tried to smooth over the difficulties that the leaked letter had caused, writing Mayor Lucas on September 16 that he had cancelled his proposed meeting with OEO leadership, and that "Tufts has no desire to control or hamper the community hospital, the town of Mound Bayou, or any other local institution." Despite James's and Maloney's conciliatory attitudes, conflict between the two institutions persisted.[35]

In the midst of this turmoil, Jack Geiger announced that he was leaving Tufts to head the brand-new Department of Community Health and Social Medicine at the State University of New York–Stony Brook. His pending departure, combined with Dean Maloney's letter critical of the situation in Mound Bayou, raised the question of what role, if any, Tufts University would continue to have in Mound Bayou, and what would happen to the health center. Geiger's decision was not entirely a surprise; for a number of years he had been searching for additional resources for the health center, and had obtained permission from the health council and senior staff as early as 1968 to begin looking for such resources. Geiger and Hatch planned for the North Bolivar County Health Council to eventually be the governing board of the health center, a process that began in 1969 when five members of the health council were placed on the health center's Board of Directors. That year, the chairman, vice chairman, secretary, treasurer, and one member at large of the health center's board were also all members of the North Bolivar County Health Council. In 1969, OEO made funds directly available for the North Bolivar County Health Council to carry out its own programs, without prior approval from Tufts or the health center.[36]

Even though North Bolivar County Health Council's takeover as owner and operator of the health center had begun before Geiger announced he was leaving Tufts, questions still remained regarding the long-term viability of the health center. Geiger assured the health council that Tufts was still interested in funding the health center, as was SUNY–Stony Brook, but that the council should explore all other options as well. In essence, the health council faced four options in light of Geiger's move to Stony Brook: (1) continue its relationship with Tufts; (2) establish a new affiliation with Stony Brook; (3) seek an entirely different university or medical

---

[35] Cefalu, "Tufts Center, Mound Bayou hospital clash"; Letter from William F. Maloney to Earl Lucas, September 16, 1970, *JGC*.

[36] North Bolivar County Health Report, n.d. (1969?) Collection 4613, Box 42, Folder 310, *DHC*, Southern Historical Collection; Dittmer, *The Good Doctors*, 234; Geiger, "A Health Center for Social Change: People and Poverty in Rural Mississippi"; Geiger, "Chronology of Conflict in Mound Bayou," *JGC*.

center sponsor; (4) apply directly to OEO without a medical school or medical center sponsor.[37]

What then transpired were a series of "reverse site visits," whereby the members of the North Bolivar County Health Council met with the administrations at Tufts, Stony Brook, Meharry, Tuskegee University, and the University of Wisconsin—all of which were interested in partnering with the health center—in order to see which institution would offer the best package to fit the needs of the people of north Bolivar County, including financial resources for the health center, academic scholarships for local residents, and the commitment of university funds for other forms of community improvement. (In addition to these schools, the Matthew Walker Health Center of Nashville, the Alto Park Neighborhood Health Center of Chattanooga, Tennessee, and the Southside Comprehensive Health Center of Atlanta, Georgia, were also all visited by representatives of the health council.) This process of a local health council making reverse site visits was unprecedented in the community health center movement and a prime example of the control that the local population—the poor of north Bolivar County—had in the decision-making process of the health center.[38]

To help reach a decision as to whom to partner with, members of the health council solicited advice from a number of community organizations and leaders, including the Delta Ministry, and established five study groups, each composed of health council members, senior staff of the health center, representatives from the Mound Bayou Community Hospital, and representatives of the town of Mound Bayou.[39]

After much contentious debate, the North Bolivar County Health Council eventually chose to follow Geiger to Stony Brook, which offered more than a dozen scholarships to Bolivar County residents as part of its proposal. The decision proved controversial, and many of Geiger's old foes criticized the council's decision. The Mound Bayou *Voice* stated that "the chief reason for deciding to affiliate with Stony Brook was that the boss, Dr. H. Jack Geiger, went there and he wanted to change the Center's affiliation to Stony Brook." The paper asserted that the University of Wisconsin offered vastly more resources.[40]

With the transition to Stony Brook, the North Bolivar County Health Council received more control over the daily operations at the health center, including the

[37] North Bolivar County Health Report, n.d. (1969?) Collection 4613, Box 42, Folder 310, *DHC*, Southern Historical Collection; Dittmer, *The Good Doctors*, 234; Geiger, "A Health Center for Social Change: People and Poverty in Rural Mississippi"; Geiger, "Chronology of Conflict in Mound Bayou," *JGC*.

[38] H. Jack Geiger, "Chronology of Conflict in Mound Bayou," *JGC*; "Stony Brook Chosen as University Affiliate," *Compared to What?: The TUFTS–Delta Health Center Newsletter* (January 1971), Box 20, Folder 149, *DHC*.

[39] Stony Brook Chosen as University Affiliate," *Compared to What?: The TUFTS–Delta Health Center Newsletter* (January 1971), Box 20, Folder 149, *DHC*.

[40] "Stony Brook Chosen as University Affiliate," *Compared to What?: The TUFTS–Delta Health Center Newsletter* (January 1971), Box 20, Folder 149, *DHC*; "N.B.C. Health Council 'Decision' to Hurt Poor," *The Voice* [Mound Bayou, Miss.], Jan. 17–30, 1971.

hiring of staff—an issue that had been a long-simmering source of conflict, because some members of the health council believed that rural residents had been passed over regularly for jobs at the health center. The health council's functions, therefore, included screening and approving applicants for positions at the center; monitoring the administration of all health services; hiring staff for support services such as transportation and day care; and maintaining the outreach facilities of the local health associations. The health council's employees answered only to the board, and council decisions were accepted both by university administrators and center staff as the final voice on local issues. Finally, on September 1, 1971, complete control of the center, now renamed the Delta Health Center, passed to North Bolivar County Health and Civic Improvement, Inc.[41]

The health council's control of the health center was brief, however. Even before the final agreements with Stony Brook had been signed, there was again a push, led by Mayor Earl Lucas, to consolidate the health center with the hospital under the control of a new board led by members from Mound Bayou. Lucas lobbied Dr. E. Leon Cooper, the new director of OEO's Office of Health Affairs, to give the town control over the health center and the hospital. The old arguments that the Delta Health Center and the Mound Bayou Community Hospital were providing redundant services at unnecessary costs were presented anew, and the black leaders of Mound Bayou were joined again by their unlikely political allies, including the governor of Mississippi, in pushing for a change in the OEO grant to the health center and hospital. The Nixon administration had begun to phase out OEO by 1971, converting much of its funding to block grants for the states or transferring it to other government agencies; as Greta DeJong observed, "Restoring control to Mound Bayou's administrators was politically appealing [to Nixon] because it allowed the president to make points with the advocates of greater black autonomy even as he appeased conservative southern supporters who expected action on election promises to roll back Federal interference in their states."[42]

Long resentful of Tufts's (and then Stony Brook's) control of the health center's grants, both local Mound Bayou and Mississippi state officials, albeit for vastly different reasons, pushed for the consolidation of the health center and the hospital with control of the new entity to be administered by locals. James Bivins, who later became director of the Delta Health Center, complained, "With OEO, poor people

---

[41] John Hatch, "North Bolivar County farm cooperative self-help nutritional program grant proposal, 1972," *JHC*; DeJong, "Plantation Politics, 269–70; Geiger, "A Health Center for Social Change: People and Poverty in Rural Mississippi."

[42] Huttie, "New Federalism and the Death of a Dream in Mound Bayou, Mississippi," 22; Sobleson, "Participation, Power, and Place," 83–84; DeJong, "Plantation Politics," 271–72.

had control over budgets and federal programs at the state level. What Nixon is talking about now is giving local politicians those same funds and letting them decide whether or not to continue programs like ours." In January 1972 OEO, which by then was no longer staffed with any of the health center's longtime allies, ordered the Mound Bayou Community Hospital and the Delta Health Center to combine their operations under a single OEO grant and expand services for the poor to a four-county area in the Mississippi Delta. The merged facility, which the North Bolivar County Health Council reluctantly agreed to in April, realizing that it was the only way to keep federal funding, was to be managed by a new board made up of members from the hospital's board, the health council, and the health center's board. DeJong described this as "power passed from the rural poor clientele to middle-class administrators," which in Mound Bayou meant "politicians and business leaders appointed to represent specific interests. No mechanism was created to ensure democratic participation by program recipients."[43] The board was headed by the Delta Ministry's Owen Brooks, and the organization was unaffiliated with any academic institution, just as Mound Bayou's local establishment had wanted for years.

Their realized dream soon turned to a nightmare as the new OEO grant for the merged facility was immediately vetoed by the Mississippi governor—and previous ally to the local cause—William Waller. Since its inception, the health center's federal funding had been protected from interference from Mississippi politicians because of its affiliation with an academic instruction, which, under OEO guidelines, prevented state governments from blocking the grants. Without an academic sponsor, Waller took the opportunity to try to kill the health center that he and other Mississippi politicians had opposed for years. Waller asserted that he vetoed the $5.5 million grant because the hospital did not comply with fire and building codes; that the merged facility could not serve the needs of the people; that the facilities duplicated services of other federal agencies in Mississippi; and, that since the merger already had taken place, the hospital's state license was invalid. The veto, however, was certainly little more than a spiteful attempt by the white power structure in Mississippi to rid itself of a federally funded program that it had always opposed because it benefitted—and empowered—the state's black citizens.[44]

The governor's veto put the health care of indigent blacks in Bolivar County into immediate crisis. Dr. Thomas Gualtieri, the director of the merged facilities, now known as the Delta Community Hospital and Health Center, Inc., told *The New York Times* in the summer of 1972, "Unless we get some help in the next week or two, will have to cut medical services drastically. People will not get medicine.

---

[43] DeJong, "Plantation Politics," 273–74.
[44] "Mound Bayou Hospitals: Veto halts merger," *Delta Democrat-Times*, June 18, 1972.

Some will get sick, some will die." Staff at the hospital and health center worked for weeks without pay while the grant was in limbo, with some of the staff joining their patients on the welfare rolls. The decision of Mississippi's governor to block federal funding for health programs for indigent blacks made national news—the issue of OEO funding for the Delta Community Hospital and Health Center even came to the floor of the 1972 Democratic National Convention—and Waller eventually approved the grant. Despite the fact that the Delta Hospital and Health Center eventually got the grant, Joseph Huttie argued that "the fact that OEO, locked in its own death struggle with the Nixon administration, felt the need to negotiate with the governor was a strong indication of the President's determination to gut most federal programs controlled and managed by the poor themselves."[45]

By 1972, the Tufts–Delta Health Center, as initially created and envisioned, ceased to exist. All of its founding figures—Jack Geiger, John Hatch, Bob Smith, Aaron Shirley, L. C. Dorsey, and Andrew James—had left Mound Bayou, having moved on to new challenges, and the center's medical school affiliations were also history. Although the health center never closed its doors or stopped providing care for the poor of north Bolivar County, the merged Delta Community Hospital and Health Center, Inc., now operated under the control of a new board, run primarily by the city leaders of Mound Bayou, and much of its original mission had changed. With much of the Great Society to be dismantled in the 1970s, the Delta Community Hospital and Health Center, Inc., faced enormous challenges ahead.

[45] Roy Reed, "Political Dispute Perils Funds for Mississippi Health Facility," *The New York Times,* July 17, 1972; "Waller OK's Health Grant; Calls Bayou Project 'Fiasco,'" *Memphis Commercial Appeal,* July 8, 1972; Huttie, "New Federalism and the Death of a Dream in Mound Bayou, Mississippi," 23.

I just wanted to put my education to use and help people.
DR. ANDREW JAMES

7

Epilogue

IN THE SUMMER of 2014, fifty years after Lyndon Johnson proclaimed a War on Poverty, the brand new 26,000-square-foot, $5 million Dr. H. Jack Geiger Medical Center at the Delta Health Center was dedicated in Mound Bayou. The previous health center building was renamed for Drs. John Hatch and Andrew James, and repurposed for educational programs. A year earlier, Jack Geiger, L. C. Dorsey, Andy James, John Hatch, Helen Barnes, Bob Smith, Aaron Shirley, Willie Lucas, and a host of other figures from the early years of the Tufts–Delta Health Center came together to break ground on the new building. Many of them returned for the opening of the new facility, but some were absent, most notably L. C. Dorsey, who passed away in 2013. In addition to the new Dr. H. Jack Geiger Medical Center in Mound Bayou, in 2015 the Delta Health Center also operated a separate dental clinic in Mound Bayou and satellite facilities in Cleveland, Indianola, and Moorhead, with two in Greenville.

In the more than four decades since they left Mound Bayou, the center these men and women founded and nurtured in the late-1960s and early-1970s went through a series of crises—both financial and administrative—but has continued to provide, as its slogan states, "Health Care with Care." The Delta Health Center is a continuing legacy of one of the many often unknown, or underappreciated, successes of Lyndon Johnson's Great Society. Today, the Delta Health Center is one of more than 1,200 community health centers in the United States that deliver care at over

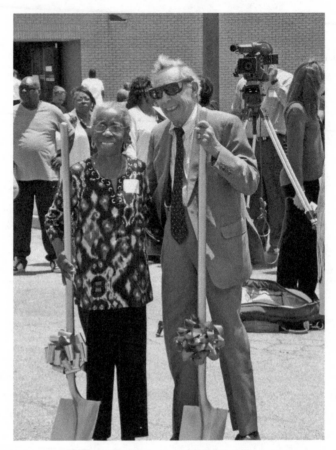

FIGURE 7.1 L.C. Dorsey and Jack Geiger at the groundbreaking ceremony for the Dr. H. Jack
Geiger Medical Center at the Delta Health Center in 2013 (photo credit: Tom Ward).

9,000 sites across the nation. The Community Health Center Program, of which the
Tufts–Delta Health Center and Columbia Point were the forerunners, is the largest
primary-care medical network in the United States, serving more than 28 million
low-income patients a year in 2015, more than 72 percent of whom lived below the
federal poverty line.[1] Community health centers operate in every state in the union,
in rural and urban areas, and there are health centers that serve specific populations, such as migrant workers, high school students, and public housing residents.
Federal grants provide only a portion of the funding for community health centers;
the rest is paid for by patients through Medicare and Medicaid, private insurance,

---

[1] National Association of Community Health Centers, "United States Health Center Fact Sheet" (https://
www.nachc.com/client/documents/America's_CHCs1014.pdf); Annelise Orleck and Lisa Gayle Hazirjian,
Eds., *The War on Poverty: A New Grassroots History, 1964–1980* (Athens and London: University of Georgia
Press, 2011): 440.

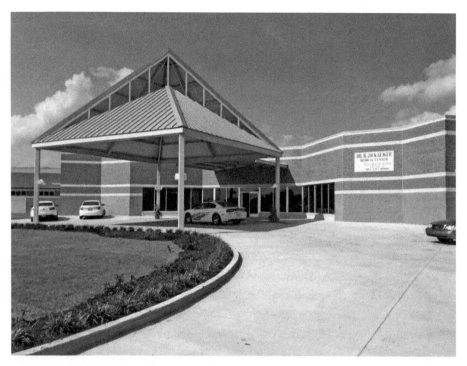

FIGURE 7.2 The Dr. H. Jack Geiger Medical Center of the Delta Health Center, Mound Bayou, Mississippi, opened 2014 (photo credit: Tom Ward).

or self-pay on a sliding scale based on income for those without insurance, although no one is turned away for lack of insurance or ability to pay. Community health centers, along with Medicare and Medicaid, have done more to improve the health of America's poor over the past half century than any other program, public or private; they are one of the great achievements and legacies of the War on Poverty.

* * *

In the early-1970s, following the departure of many of its founding members and the transfer of the federal grant to its newly minted board, the now-combined Delta Community Hospital and Health Center (DCHHC) faced a number of immediate crises. The first, Governor Waller's veto of the grant, was eventually resolved through political channels, but the release of federal funds, although necessary to the survival of the center and hospital, did not solve all of its problems.

By 1971–1972 there were "some second-wave problems," as Geiger described them. "John Hatch had left to go to Chapel Hill and earn his doctorate. Jim Taylor and other people in community health action had left. There had been substantial turnover among the physicians. It was too soon for people who were in [professional] training from here to be back." Professional staffing, which always had been a difficult issue for both the hospital and health center, became even more challenging after the loss of outside academic sponsors. Although Meharry maintained its long-standing program of sending residents to the Mound Bayou hospital, without Tufts's (and, to a lesser extent, Stony Brook's) sponsorship, attracting qualified personnel to rural Mississippi became increasingly difficult. "There was no real thought of how all of this would get staffed without a medical school affiliation and connections," reflected Geiger. "In the main, we didn't take faculty from . . . Tufts Medical School and bring them down here, but people who came got Tufts Medical School faculty appointments, which was an enormously important recruiting reward. We negotiated that the people who were here, through Tufts as well as others, would stay on for at least a while." Later, without the carrot of faculty appointments at prestigious medical schools like Tufts and Stony Brook, relocating to Mound Bayou was an increasingly tough sell to qualified medical professionals.[2]

The crisis in professional staffing came to a head in the fall of 1972 when four of the health center's physicians sent a letter to the American Public Health Association (APHA), which had been tasked with investigating the Delta Hospital and Health Center in response to the claims made by Mississippi's governor when he vetoed the OEO grant. "We are all dealing," they wrote, "with an issue of paramount importance: The health and well-being of human beings in the Mississippi Delta." The four doctors feared that the merger was going to bring an end to the good works that the health center had been doing, and urged the APHA to recommend that the new entity be placed under a new administration and board, because, they wrote, "the present administration is simply not competent to deal with pressing issues of health and health care delivery; and that the present board is neither representative of our community nor competent to carry out its wishes." Furthermore, the doctors asserted that the current board was "dedicated to making jobs, [not] to the urgent needs of the people." Because of the turmoil with the new board, one of the center's physicians already had left, and four of the center's remaining five physicians were making plans to leave Mound Bayou. "We are leaving only with the greatest reluctance," the physicians stated. "We are leaving, not out of personal considerations. . . . Rather, we leave because, in attempting to practice good medicine, we have been stretched to the limits of endurance; not out of circumstance, but out of problems created by the project itself."[3]

By early 1973 there were only three physicians left on the health center's staff, along with two others at the hospital, and Owen Brooks, then board chairman of the Delta Community Hospital and Health Center, lamented to *Jet* magazine that,

---

[2] Geiger interview with Korstad and Boothby.

[3] Letter from Thomas Gualtieri, MD; Joanna Robert, MD; Frank D. Moeller, MD; and Ethelyn J. Williams, MD, to Dr. Thomas Georges and the members of the American Public Health Association Task Force, Sept. 14, 1972, Series 1, Subseries 1, Box 7, Folder 52, *DHC*.

"we need more doctors." Things had become so bad that many poor people in the area just stopped using the hospital or health center at all. It seemed like "a return to the days before the health center arrived," remarked Geiger, one in which "the people get screwed—except now it's happening to the tune of four million dollars a year." One nurse at the health center was so distraught with how things had deteriorated that she wrote a letter to the *Memphis Commercial Appeal* complaining about the new leadership and what it was doing to the center. It became known as the "Sad Nurse" letter, because the woman refused to identify herself, "out of fear for what would happen to my relatives if I did." She stated only that she was a black nurse who had worked at both the Tufts–Delta Health Center and the Mound Bayou Community Hospital for years. She said that she hoped that if her letter was published and people found out the truth about what was happening in Mound Bayou, then "health care for black people in the Delta can be saved from its real enemies, who were Owen Brooks and Earl Lucas and the whole Mound Bayou gang that will destroy it just as surely as the governor of Mississippi would."[4]

Under the new board, positions at the center were now handed out mainly through political patronage, and often even nepotism. As Geiger bitterly recalled, "They simply handed out all those senior jobs." Lucas's wife, Mary Lee, headed the nursing staff, and his brother Willie, who had received his medical degree through assistance from Jack Geiger at Tufts Medical School, served as the medical director of the Delta Community Hospital and Health Center, Inc. Another of the mayor's brothers served as director of personnel, while a sister-in-law was director of the hospital and health center's social services. L. C. Dorsey, who had left Mound Bayou in 1971 to attend Stony Brook, returned to Mississippi after completing her master's degree in social work. She hoped to continue her career at the health center, but found that "They were not hiring anybody who were identified as part of the Geiger/Hatch group. So we came back with [degrees] in hand and found ourselves totally unemployed. In my particular situation, since I'd been a civil rights activist, I couldn't find work anywhere."[5]

In the mid-1970s, both the number and quality of services provided by the Delta Community Hospital and Health Center declined dramatically. Meharry ended its residency program with the hospital in 1975, further reducing the number of trained physicians at the hospital, and many of the programs that previously had been conducted by the health center—and which had made it so effective—were reduced

---

[4] "We Need More Doctors," *Jet* (Feb. 15, 1973): 30–31; DeJong, "Plantation Politics," 274; Letter from "Sad Nurse" to Mr. A. B. Albritton, *Memphis Commercial Appeal*, July 31, 1972.

[5] Geiger interview with Ward; Rodgers, *Life and Death in the Delta*, 157–58; L. C. Dorsey interview by Korstad and Boothby.

or eliminated. "We just started to lose services until what we were all left with is almost totally the provision of health care, very little of the other support services," remembered L. C. Dorsey. "All of that, of course, can be attributed to the people in Mound Bayou who took over. It also was part of what was happening with the nation. Those things ceased to be important with the administrations that followed the Johnson administration." Most of the outreach programs at the health center were discontinued, as were education programs, youth services, food distribution, home nursing care, and the environmental health unit, as the annual federal funding for the center was reduced from $5.5 million to $3.3 million during the Nixon administration, resulting in 130 of the health center's 450-person staff being laid off. Unlike the comprehensive programs that had been hallmarks of the health center's early years, after the entire community health center program was transferred from OEO to the Department of Health, Education and Welfare (HEW) in the early 1970s, officials there restricted the health center's services to those that were deemed directly related to medical care of individual patients. "We used to be able to make attempts at cleaning up the kind of living conditions that result in the serious disease here," stated Herman Johnson, a Mound Bayou alderman and Resources Coordinator at the Health Center. We've lost our ability to prevent disease that can be prevented."[6]

From 1972 to 1984 the Delta Community Hospital and Health Center operated on federal grants, first from OEO and then HEW. During this period, health centers across the nation faced repeated opposition, then change. In 1972 HEW declared that federal support was no longer needed for community health centers, because they could collect reimbursements from Medicare, Medicaid, and private insurers; they thereby needed to be self-sufficient. The next year Nixon asked Congress to phase out the legislation under which the health centers were funded. In response, Sen. Ted Kennedy, who had been a supporter of the community health center program since its inception, introduced a bill to protect, and even strengthen, community health centers. President Gerald Ford pocket vetoed the health center legislation in 1974 and vetoed it in 1975. Congress, however, overrode the veto, and "the program emerged stronger and better defined than any time in its past," according to Bonnie Lefkowitz in *Community Health Centers: A Movement and the People Who Made it Happen.* As a result of the new legislation, the number of centers expanded significantly, from 158 in 1974 to 872 nationwide in 1980, but, wrote Lefkowitz, these centers "tended to be small, and only about 5 million people were being served in total . . . [as they] implemented

---

[6] DeJong, "Plantation Politics," 273; L. C. Dorsey interview by Korstad and Boothby; Huttie, 21, 28.

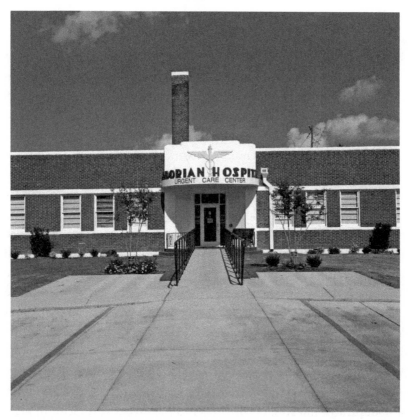

FIGURE 7.3 The Taborian Hospital Building, Mound Bayou, Mississippi. Originally constructed in 1942 by the Knights and Daughters of Tabor, it later became the Mound Bayou Community Hospital. It closed in 1983 (photo credit: Tom Ward).

a 'lean and mean' model, without most of the non-health services that character-ized the earlier grantees. Since increases in appropriations did not keep pace with the phenomenal growth rate, some of the money for expansion came from cuts in support for the older, more comprehensive centers." During his first month in office, Ronald Reagan, who declared war on the War on Poverty, proposed con-solidating eighty-eight federal programs, including community health centers, into seven block grants to states and localities. Critics argued that such block grants would eliminate or reduce funding to programs, such as community health centers, with weak political constituencies, by placing control of funds with state governors. Congress rejected the plan for block grants, but Reagan did reverse the trend of increased spending for the nation's health centers, cut-ting appropriations from $368 million in 1981 to $301 million in 1982. As a result of these cuts, 187 health centers were phased out, and most others saw reduced funding.[7]

The Delta Community Hospital, beset by administrative and financial woes, saw its patient load decline dramatically as black residents of the Delta, many now insured by Medicaid or Medicare, turned to the area's larger, more modern public hospitals, which had previously barred them. The facility, which had served black residents of the region in one form or another since its opening in 1942 as Taborian Hospital, eventually lost its state accreditation and closed its doors in 1983. The next year the HEW regional office in Atlanta informed the Delta Health Center, which earlier had received a federal grant to modernize its clinical facility, that it would be defunded and closed if it did not remove its current leadership and establish a new board of directors. HEW was especially critical of the center's large deficits, its inability to bill Medicare and Medicaid adequately, and its failure to recruit professional staff. After much turmoil, eventually a new board was created, and L. C. Dorsey—now Dr. Dorsey after earning her doctorate in social work from Howard University and a certificate in health care management form Johns Hopkins—was hired as executive director of the Delta Health Center, which she had first come to at work two decades earlier as a high school dropout and unemployed sharecropper. After spending a number of years working for criminal justice reform, in particular the treatment of death-row inmates, she began her role as executive director in 1988, and found the center to be a financial and administrative mess. "I was the seventh director in a three year period. So there had been a complete lack of stability in the program," she recalled. "There'd been a purchasing scam where people had been stealing $1 million worth of stuff, and three of them finally went to federal prison from here. There had been a lot of bad things that really made people's morale low." Under Dorsey's direction, from 1988 to 1995, the health center not only became financially stable, but was able to expand its services once again. During her tenure as director, the center's facility was enlarged and modernized, and it extended programs to neighboring Coahoma, Sunflower, and Washington counties. "When I took over most of our money was from federal grants," Dorsey stated. "By the time I left 75 percent came from Medicaid, Medicare, other insurance, and private pay patients."[8]

---

[7] Clymer, *Edward M. Kennedy*, 315–16; Lefkowitz, *Community Health Centers*, 13–16, 20. For more on the changes in federal funding for Community Health Centers in the 1970s and 1980s, see Alice Sardell, *The U.S. Experiment in Social Medicine: The Community Health Center Program, 1965–1986* (Pittsburgh, Penn.: University of Pittsburgh Press, 1988).

[8] Geiger, "Chronology of Conflict in Mound Bayou," *JGC*; L. C. Dorsey interview by Robert Korstad and Neil Boothby; Lefkowitz, *Community Health Centers*, 44–45.

The North Bolivar County Farm Cooperative, which L. C. Dorsey had been managing before she left Mississippi to further her education, also suffered in the years after Tufts left Mississippi and the co-op distanced itself from the health council. As it struggled to survive financially on its own after the loss of federal funding, the co-op faced a number of challenges, including an attempt in 1972 to take the land and turn it into a commercial fish farm. The co-op's mission, and its difficulties, inspired people from around the nation to support it with donations of cash and goods. In Massachusetts, a young mother, Kay Doherty, raised $56,600 for the co-op over a two-year period. She first became aware of the North Bolivar County Farm Cooperative in a 1972 *Boston Globe* article that described the farm and the difficulties that it faced in the wake of government cutbacks to the OEO program. "The injustices described in the article just screamed at me," she recalled. "I knew that our tax money was being spent for subsidies some wealthy people were getting not to grow anything on their land. And to see and hear that people trying to grow food to feed themselves were being cut out of the Federal budget at a time when subsidies were continued, that seemed to me morally wrong." Doherty decided to stage a twenty-mile Good Friday walk for the co-op, and asked friends and neighbors to sponsor her. She eventually got thirty other people to join her, and their Good Friday march raised $3,100 for the co-op. Inspired by her story, Davis Taylor, publisher of *The Boston Globe*, offered to fly her to Mississippi to deliver her check in person. Shocked by the poverty she found there, she returned home determined to do more to help the people of Bolivar County. She organized another Good Friday march in 1973, this time with 800 participants, and raised $16,000. The money went to purchasing forty acres of land for the farm, which became known as "Kay's 40 acres." The next year the march was even larger, with over a thousand walkers and $32,000 raised. In addition to raising funds with the Good Friday walks, Doherty collected food and clothing for the people of Bolivar County. Willie Finch, then the chairman of the farm co-op, said of Kay Doherty and her supporters, "When we were about to go under, they sent us money; when we were hungry, they sent us food. The best way we can thank them is to use the money in our effort to make ourselves self-sufficient."[9]

Despite the efforts of Kay Doherty and others, the impact of federal cuts to the co-op was devastating, and during the 1970s and 1980s it struggled to maintain its membership or produce a crop; equipment went unmaintained, and some was even stolen. John Hatch, who remained in contact with many of those in Bolivar County even after he left the health center, was troubled by what happened to the co-op that he worked so hard to make a reality. He complained that "some of the locals just

---

[9] L. C. Dorsey interview with Korstad and Boothby; Black, *People and Plows Against Hunger*, 43–50.

plain wanted to steal [the land] after we left . . . just rip it off," but that L. C. Dorsey, during her time as director of the co-op, had established that the co-op's land could never be used for profit. Today, what had been the North Bolivar County Farm Co-op is the Alcorn State University Demonstration Farm, which continues to fulfill an educational mission. There is still a small community garden on some of the land that had been the original co-op farm, but it now serves mainly people in Mound Bayou instead of the wider county.[10]

Although the co-op eventually proved to be a failed experiment, the educational programs and mentoring provided through the Tufts–Delta Health Center during the late 1960s and early 1970s proved to be its most enduring legacies. Not only did people like L. C. Dorsey and Willie Lucas have the chance to leave Mississippi for educational opportunities that they probably never would have had otherwise, but they returned to Mississippi both to make their careers and provide a second wave of leadership for the black community. Dorsey called the Tufts–Delta Health Center "the original incubator" for the development of local leaders in health care, as well as many other fields. "The most important contribution that the health center has made in Mound Bayou and in the state," she wrote, "is their investment in and nurturing local potential." Addie Peterson started as a youth worker at the health center in the 1960s and went on to become the first director of the Aaron Henry Health Center in Clarksdale, while Johnny Todd, a community organizer at the health center, became mayor of Rosedale, one of the first black elected officials in the state since Reconstruction. Andy James notes that the first licensed black sanitarians in the state were recruited and trained through the center, including James Hodges and Mitchell Williams, who now serve as Chairman of the Board and Finance Chairman, respectively, of the Delta Health Center's Board of Directors. Jack Geiger proudly recounts the educational success of the people touched by the health center and the long-term impact of the center on the Delta. "There are five black Ph.Ds from that initial area. Two Ph.D. clinical psychologists from Alligator, Mississippi, population 900. Three others in other fields. . . . There are at least seven physicians out of that initial crew. There are about fifteen social workers. There are about twelve RNs," Geiger recalled in a 1992 interview. "That's all a consequence in the main of our original intervention. . . . The role models, the assistance, and the experience with black health professionals that many people had not seen earlier made a difference. . . . Directly or indirectly, this has made a difference in terms of the educational aspirations and educational achievement of people. For the longer term, that may be one of the most important consequences of this intervention."[11]

---

[10] Ward interview with Hatch and Geiger.
[11] Dorsey, "Dirt Dauber Nests"; Geiger interview with Korstad and Boothby.

In addition to those who came up through programs at the health center, those who worked there during its formative years also went on to do a number of remarkable things. Andrew James earned his Ph.D. in environmental science and became chair of the Health Services Administration at the College of Pharmacy and Health Sciences at Texas Southern University. John Hatch earned his doctorate in public health from the University of North Carolina at Chapel Hill, where he then served as a professor in the School of Public Health until his retirement, becoming the first African American in UNC's history to be appointed to a distinguished endowed chair. At Chapel Hill, Hatch expanded the recruitment of poor and black students, and trained a number of South African students who returned to senior government health positions in post-apartheid South Africa. Hatch also taught at the City College of New York Medical School and served as the project director of the health education project in Cameroon. In 1984 he was appointed to the board of the Christian Medical Council of the World Council of Churches, headquartered in Geneva, Switzerland. Dr. Robert Smith remained in Mississippi, keeping a private practice in Jackson but remaining active in the community health movement, eventually opening Central Mississippi Health Services, a community health center in Jackson. He still serves on the board of directors of the Mississippi Primary Health Care Association, which represents the state's twenty-one community health care centers, some of which were established by other physicians who had served for a time at the Tufts–Delta Health Center. Dr. Helen Barnes also remained in Mississippi, spending the bulk of her career at the University of Mississippi Medical Center, where, as an associate professor of obstetrics and gynecology, she became the school's first black faculty member.

Inspired by the model of the Tufts–Delta Health Center, Dr. Aaron Shirley committed himself to opening a similar facility in his hometown of Jackson. Partnering with other physicians, Shirley applied for an OEO grant to open a community health center. "We asked Jack Geiger to help us put together an application for here [in Jackson], and he did," remembered Shirley. As it had in the Delta, opposition to the proposed center manifested from among local politicians and doctors; however, unlike in Mound Bayou, Shirley did not have a university sponsor, and the OEO grant quickly was vetoed by the governor. After an appeal to then OEO director Donald Rumsfeld, the governor's veto was overturned and the grant was funded. With the grant, Shirley and his partners established the Jackson–Hinds Health Center in 1970, which, like the Tufts–Delta Health Center, provided comprehensive health services for the poor in the Jackson area, including environmental services, mental health programs, housing for senior citizens, and counseling for teenagers. Shirley also promoted civic responsibility, encouraging patients to register and vote. By 1979 Jackson–Hinds was the largest community health center in the state and a model for health centers nationwide. In 1993 Shirley received a MacArthur Foundation "genius award," which he used to help convert a derelict shopping center into the Jackson Medical Mall. After raising over $20 million to renovate the space, and partnering with a number of the state's institutions of higher learning, the Medical Mall now houses numerous clinics, medical support firms, offices, classrooms, and retail outlets. It was the first facility of its kind and serves as a model for similar developments in other cities. Because of his innovative contributions in medical care, Shirley was invited to serve as a health policy advisor to President Bill Clinton, and in 2005 the University of Mississippi Medical Center established an endowed chair in his name. In 2010, in a return to the practices of the Tufts–Delta Health Center's early years, Shirley created HealthConnect, a program using door-to-door community health workers to educate the poor about preventing the diseases borne out of poverty and obesity.[12]

After leaving Mound Bayou, Jack Geiger directed the Department of Community Medicine at SUNY–Stony Brook until 1978, when he was offered an endowed chair to establish the Department of Community Health and Social Medicine at the City University of New York Medical School in Harlem, which specifically focused on recruiting students from underrepresented minorities and impoverished communities. Students were admitted out of high school into the combined undergraduate–graduate program, which culminated with an M.D. To pay for their state-subsidized education, these newly minted physicians agreed to practice for a time in poor and underserved communities. Both John Hatch and Sydney Kark were brought in as visiting professors during Geiger's almost two decades leading the program at the City University of New York. Geiger retired in 1998, but continued teaching and lecturing at the school as the Arthur C. Logan Professor Emeritus of Community Medicine.

In addition to his work at the City University of New York, Geiger remained active in his lifelong pursuit of public health and civil rights. He was a founding member and president of Physicians for Social Responsibility, the antinuclear organization that shared the 1986 Nobel Peace Prize. That year he helped found Physicians for Human Rights, which also shared the Nobel Peace Prize in 1998 for its humanitarian and healthcare missions to the West Bank and Gaza Strip; to Bosnia, Croatia, Serbia, and Kosovo during the Balkan Wars; and to Iraq following the first Gulf War. Geiger returned to South Africa on a number of occasions, often with John Hatch, and in 1995 spent several months as a Distinguished Visiting Professor at the

---

[12] Dittmer, *The Good Doctors*, 280–81; Lefkowitz, *Community Health Centers*, 40; Jimmie E. Gates, "Medical Pioneer Dr. Aaron Shirley Has Died," *Jackson Clarion-Ledger* (November 27, 2014); Suzy Hansen, "What Can Mississippi Learn from Iran?" *The New York Times*, July 27, 2012.

University of Natal Medical School in Durban, where he had first come as a visiting medical student to study community health centers in 1957. Geiger also served as a consultant to South Africa's Truth and Reconciliation Commission. In 1998 he was awarded the highest honor of the Institute of Medicine, the Gustav O. Lienhard Award, for his community health center work and for "outstanding contributions to minority health," and he received the American Public Health Association's highest honor, the Sedgwick Memorial Medal, for his decades of work for civil rights and public health. After years of estrangement from the Delta Health Center, Geiger again became involved with the center as a consultant once L. C. Dorsey became its director in 1988, an association that continues to this day.

* * *

The Affordable Care Act (ACA), or Obamacare, faced many of the same criticisms that the community health centers withstood when they were established in the 1960s. The cries of "socialized medicine" that Jack Geiger heard from Mississippi physicians and politicians echoed loudly in the recent debates surrounding the Affordable Care Act. Although much of the discussion of the ACA has focused on the individual mandate for purchasing health insurance, the law also provides for a substantial investment in the nation's community health centers as a means of delivering care to the nation's poor. The ACA provides over $11 billion over its first five years for the operation, expansion, and construction of community health centers in the United States. This increased funding for community health centers already has expanded the number of people in the country who have access to health care. It is also central to lowering health care costs, as numerous studies have shown that increases in preventive care coincide with decreases in expensive emergency room visits in communities with access to community health centers.[13] The impact of community health centers around the nation far outweighs their costs, not only in the services that they provide to their communities, but also in their economic impact. As in Bolivar County, where the economic impact of the Delta Health Center was, and continues to be, significant, community health centers nationwide generated over $20 billion in economic activity for low-income communities in 2009, a figure that is expected to rise to over $50 billion by 2015, with the expansion of centers and services under the ACA.[14]

Unfortunately, in Mississippi, despite the fact that there are now twenty-one community health centers throughout the state, each of which also operates numerous satellite facilities, health care for the state's poorest citizens remains woefully

---

[13] Health Resources & Services Administration Fact Sheet (http://bphc.hrsa.gov/about/healthcenterfactsheet.pdf); Mississippi Primary Health Care Association, " Community Health Centers Directory of Services, 2011," (www.mphca.com/313047+MPHCA-Directory+of+Services+2011.pdf)

[14] Mississippi Primary Health Care Association, "Community Health Centers Directory of Services, 2011."

inadequate. The average black man in Mississippi has a shorter life expectancy than the average American had in 1960. Sixty-nine percent of adult Mississippians are over-weight, because many live in "food deserts" and do not have access to healthy food. Consequently, Mississippians are dying from diabetes, hypertension, congestive heart disease, and asthma at higher rates than the nation as a whole. Aaron Shirley remarked that in the 1960s people in Mississippi starved, but today they die from food. Because of the intransigence of the Republican governor of Mississippi, Phil Bryant, regard-ing the expansion of Medicaid in the state, Mississippi is the only state in the union where the percentage of uninsured residents actually increased since the implemen-tation of the Affordable Care Act. Bryant's refusal, along with the vast majority of Republican governors nationwide, to participate in the federal government's Medicaid expansion—which would have initially cost the state nothing—left over 138,000 poor Mississippians, most of whom are black, with no insurance. Without the expansion, Mississippi's Medicaid program is one of the most restrictive in the nation, excluding all able-bodied adults without children, and only permitting families who earn less than 22 percent of the federal poverty level—less than $400 a month—to enroll. As a result, Mississippi remains at or near the bottom of almost all health statistics in the nation.[15]

* * *

Despite Ronald Reagan's infamous statement, "In the sixties we waged a war on pov-erty, and poverty won," in many ways, most Great Society programs did not fail, as much as they were cut off at the knees and forced to move away from their roots. In fact, despite public perception, poverty decreased substantially as a result of the programs of the Great Society. Between 1964 and 1974, the number of Americans living in poverty was cut in half, from 22 percent to 11 percent, and the number of the nation's children living in poverty dropped from 27 percent to 14 percent. Funding cuts in the 1970s and 1980s, however, destroyed many War on Poverty programs and left others, including community health centers, economically devastated. Poverty rates began to creep back up. Because of both funding cuts and ineffective leadership, much of the radical experimentation of the original Tufts–Delta Health Center, which focused on the question of "What does it take to be healthy and stay healthy, not just get healthy?" was abandoned in the 1970s and 1980s for a leaner community health care model. "Once the programs were transferred to HEW the purpose was lost on innovation," recalled OEO Senior Program Analyst Ann Haendel. "They are

---

[15] Hansen, "What Can Mississippi Learn from Iran?"; Sarah Varney, "How Obamacare Went South in Mississippi," *Kaiser Health News,* October 29, 2014 (http://khn.org/news/how-obamacare-went-south-in-mississippi/). Varney's article provides a fascinating—and disturbing—insight into how and why the ACA has failed in Mississippi, and its impact on the poor there.

not family centered, we don't have the community involvement to the same degree." Geiger lamented that, as a result of federal cuts in the 1980s, the services at community health centers across the nation were forced to adopt a more limited "market model" of health care that focused almost entirely on clinical care, abandoning much of the focus on preventative care, public health, outreach, and educational programs that were the hallmarks of the Tufts–Delta Health Center. Community health centers became "federally funded Medicaid mills urged to be lean, mean and competitive—as if anybody were competing to take care of these populations," remarked Geiger in a 1992 interview. "There is little conception of the vision of health services and health interventions that had existed before."[16] There has been renewed interest in the past few years at the Delta Health Center to return to some of the practices of the original Tufts–Delta Health Center, to understand the social determinants of health. For example, a community garden has been planted on health center grounds in recent years, where a variety of vegetables are grown and are free to those who want to come pick them. There is also a renewed focus on preventive care, including teaching people the importance of exercise and eating fresh fruits and vegetables. Finally, there also has been a return to an emphasis on educational programs at the center.

Critics often point to the fact that many War on Poverty programs, like the Delta Health Center, survived only through government aid, and were never self-supporting entities. This is true, but the argument ignores both the direct and indirect impact of such programs on the communities they served—and still serve. Although the programs of the health center were funded by government money, it was not a handout, but an opportunity. "It gave numerous people jobs. It put a lot back into the community," remembered Barbara Brooks, who worked at the health center in the 1960s. "Gave a lot of people self-esteem. It also educated people—they sent us to school if you wanted to go to school. They set up programs for the illiterate peoples, those that could not read, they tried to help them to do that, and to show them that they had nothing to be ashamed of. It taught people how to take seeds and grow and develop those seeds, and tomato plants and what they needed to do in order to make it work, to fertilize it, to cultivate it." These programs have proven to be economically positive not only for the communities they serve, but for taxpayers as well, because for every $1 million in federal funding invested in community health centers, $1.73 million in jobs and increased economic activity is created.[17]

---

[16] Annelise Orleck, "Introduction: The War on Poverty from the Grass Roots Up," in Annelise Orleck and Lisa Gayle Hazirjian, Eds., *The War on Poverty: A New Grassroots History, 1964–1980* (Athens and London: University of Georgia Press, 2011), 6–7; Sobelson, "Participation, Power, and Place," 93; Ward interview with Ann Haendel; Geiger interview with Korstad and Boothby.

[17] Interview with Barbara Brooks and Jack Cartwright; Mississippi Primary Health Care Association, "Community Health Centers Directory of Services, 2011."

The legacy of the Tufts–Delta Health Center is therefore much more than the medical care that it delivered to thousands of desperately poor people, although that care was certainly not insignificant. In both practical and symbolic terms, the Tufts–Delta Health Center was a radical assault on both the medical and the social status quo, which is why it faced so much opposition from so many fronts. As part of the Great Society, and its federal funding, it challenged the local control and "states' rights" philosophy dominant in Mississippi and throughout the South. With its innovations in healthcare delivery, its emphasis on the social determinants of health—including education, preventative care, nutrition, and the environment—the center upended traditional approaches to medical care. Most importantly, as it emerged out of the civil rights movement, it challenged the racial, social, and class systems of Mississippi with its mission to empower the poor and dispossessed through community engagement. As Dr. Aaron Shirley, who passed away in 2014, remarked,

And now, I realize, it was that element that those who resisted were most threatened by, not just the medical. The medical piece threatened the establishment to the degree that it would expose the traditional system for what it was, and it really wasn't making a difference, and it really did nothing to narrow the gap between health stats. The exposure of all of these medical conditions at a time where they should not have existed, but did. But the other piece was more threatening in terms of change, social change.[18]

---

[18] Aaron Shirley interview.

BIBLIOGRAPHY

MANUSCRIPT COLLECTIONS

Meharry Medical College Archives, Nashville, Tennessee

Matthew Walker Papers

Mississippi Department of Archives and History, Jackson, Mississippi

Mississippi Sovereignty Commission files. Sovereignty Commission Online. http://mdah.state.
ms.us/arrec/digital_archives/sovcom/

Moorland–Spingarn Research Center, Howard University, Washington, D.C.

Dorothy Ferebee Papers

Special Collections, Mitchell Library, Mississippi State University, Starkville, Mississippi

John C. Stennis Collection
Tombigbee Council on Human Relations Collection

Private (in possession of the author)

L. C. Dorsey Collection
John Hatch Collection
Jack Geiger Collection

Southern Historical Collection, Wilson Library, University of North Carolina–Chapel Hill

Delta Health Center Records, 1956–1992. Collection 4613.
John Hatch Papers, 1967–1995. Collection 04801.

Wisconsin Historical Society Archives, Madison, Wisconsin

North Bolivar County Farm Co-op Records
Lee Bankhead Papers

ORAL HISTORIES

* * *

Delta Health Center Tapes (in possession of the author)

Interview with John Hatch, Delta Health Center Tapes, Disk 1, Reel 5–2.
Interview with Andy James, Delta Health Center Tapes, Disk 1, Reel 5–5.
Mrs. Clementine Murray Interview, Delta Health Center Tapes, Disk 1, Reels 5–6 & 5–7.
Angetta Soderberg Interview, Delta Health Center Tapes, Disk 1, Reel 5–8.
Mrs. White Oral History, Delta Health Center Tapes, Disk 1, Reel 5–9.
L. C. Dorsey Interview, Delta Health Center Tapes, Disk 1, Reel 5–1.
Mrs. Lucinda Young Oral History, Delta Health Center Tapes, Disk 1, Reel 5–10.

Southern Historical Collection, University of North Carolina at Chapel Hill

Interview with Barbara Brooks and Jack Cartwright by Martha Minette in Rosedale, Mississippi, 1999.
Interview with John Brown by John Hatch.
Interview with Mayor Earl Lewis.
Interview with Dr. Aaron Shirley by Dr. John Hatch, July 18, 1992.
Interview with Rev. H. Y. Ward by John Hatch.

Southern Rural Poverty Collection, Duke University

Interview with L. C. Dorsey by Robert Korstad and Neil Boothby, April 22, 1992. Southern Rural Poverty Collection. http://dewitt.sanford.duke.edu/wp-content/uploads/2011/09/DORSEY1.pdf.
Interview with H. Jack Geiger by Robert Korstad and Neil Boothby, April 22, 1992, Southern Rural Poverty Collection. http://dewitt.sanford.duke.edu/wp-content/uploads/2011/09/GEIGER.pdf.
Interview with John Hatch by Robert Korstad and Neil Boothby, May 26, 1992. Southern Rural Poverty Collection. http://dewitt.sanford.duke.edu/wp-content/uploads/2011/09/HATCH1.pdf.

Tougaloo College

"An interview with Robert Smith, M.D." Interviewed by Harriet Tanzman, Tougaloo College Archives, 2000.

Interviews by the Author

Sarah Atkinson, January 16, 2013.

Dr. Helen Barns, August 25, 2015.

Ann Haendel, June 17, 2013.

Drs. John Hatch and Jack Geiger, June 27, 2012.

Dr. Andrew James, June 8, 2013.

Dr. Robert Smith, June 8, 2013.

BOOKS

Asch, Chris Meyers. *The Senator and the Sharecropper: The Freedom Struggles of James O. Eastland & Fannie Lou Hamer.* New York and London: The New Press, 2008.

Beito, David T. *Black Maverick: T.R.M. Howard's Fight for Civil Rights and Economic Power.* Urbana and Chicago: University of Illinois Press, 2009.

Beito, David T. *From Mutual Aid to the Welfare State.* Chapel Hill, N.C. and London: University of North Carolina Press, 2000.

Black, Herbert. *People and Plows Against Hunger: Self-Help Experiment in a Rural Community.* Boston: Marlborough House, Inc., 1975.

Clymer, Adam. *Edward M. Kennedy: A Biography.* New York: Harper Perennial, 2000; rpr., 2009.

Cobb, James C. *The Most Southern Place on Earth.* New York: Oxford University Press, 1992.

Dittmer, John. *The Good Doctors: The Medical Committee for Human Rights and the Struggle for Social Justice in Health Care.* New York: Bloomsbury, 2009.

DeJong, Greta. "Plantation Politics: The Tufts–Delta Health Center and Interracial Class Conflict in Mississippi, 1965–1972," in Annelise Orleck and Lisa Gayle Hazirjian, Eds., *The War on Poverty: A New Grassroots History.* Athens: University of Georgia Press, 2011: 256–279.

Dorsey, L. C. *Freedom Came to Mississippi.* New York: The Field Foundation, 1977.

Gamble, Vanessa Northington. *Making a Place for Ourselves.* New York: Oxford University Press, 1995.

Gillette, Michael L. *Launching the War on Poverty: An Oral History.* New York: Oxford University Press, 2010.

Hansen, Christian M. *In the Name of the Children: The Life Story of a Pediatrician to the Poor.* Ipswich, Mass.: Roger Warner, 2005.

Hollister, Robert M., Bernard M. Kramer, and Seymour S. Bellin Eds. *Neighborhood Health Centers.* Lexington, Mass.: D.C. Health and Co., 1974.

Ivester, Jo. *The Outskirts of Hope: A Memoir of the 1960s Deep South.* Berkeley, Calif.: She Writes Press, 2015.

Kark, Sidney and Emily. *Promoting Community Health: From Pholela to Jerusalem.* Johannesburg, South Africa: Witwatersrand University Press, 1999.

Lefkowitz, Bonnie. *Community Health Centers: A Movement and the People Who Made It Happen.* New Brunswick, N.J.: Rutgers University Press, 2007.

McMillen, Neil R. *Dark Journey: Black Mississippians in the Age of Jim Crow.* Urbana and Chicago: University of Illinois Press, 1989.

Morais, Herbert M., Ed., *The History of the Afro-American in Medicine*. Cornwell Heights, Pa.: The Publisher's Agency, 1978.

The Mound Bayou Mississippi Story [pamphlet created by The Delta Center for Culture and Learning at Delta State University, n.d.].

Newman, Mark. *Divine Agitators: The Delta Ministry and Civil Rights in Mississippi*. Athens: University of Georgia Press, 2004.

Orleck, Annelise, and Lisa Gayle Hazirjian, Eds. *The War on Poverty: A New Grassroots History*. Athens: University of Georgia Press, 2011.

Percy, William Alexander. *Lanterns on the Levee: Recollections of a Planter's Son*. Alfred A. Knopf, 1941; rpr., LSU Press, 1994.

Rodgers, Kim Lacy. *Life and Death in the Delta*. New York: Palgrave MacMillan, 2006.

Sardell, Alice. *The U.S. Experiment in Social Medicine: The Community Health Center Program, 1965–1986*. Pittsburgh, Pa.: University of Pittsburg Press, 1988.

Secundy, Marion Gray, Ed., *Bioethics Research Concerns and Directions for African-Americans*. Jackson, Miss.: Tuskegee University, 2000.

Simpson, Sister Mary Stella. *Sister Stella's Babies*. New York: American Journal of Nursing Company Educational Services Division, 1978.

Stossel, Scott. *Sarge: The Life and Times of Sargent Shriver*. Washington, D.C.: Smithsonian Books, 2004.

Summerville, James. *Educating Black Doctors: A History of Meharry Medical College*. Tuscaloosa: University of Alabama Press, 1983.

Ward, Thomas J. Jr. *Black Physicians in the Jim Crow South*. Fayetteville: University of Arkansas Press, 2003.

Washington, Harriet A. *Medical Apartheid*. New York: Doubleday, 2006.

Willis, John C. *Forgotten Time: The Yazoo–Mississippi Delta After the Civil War*. Charlottesville and London: University Press of Virginia, 2000.

Wright, George C. *A History of Blacks in Kentucky, Volume 2: In Pursuit of Equality, 1890–1980*. Frankfort: Kentucky Historical Society, 2001.

Zeigler, Edward, and Susan Muenchow. *Head Start*. New York: Basic Books, 1992.

Ziegler, Edward, and Sally J. Styfco, Eds. *Head Start and Beyond*. New Haven and London: Yale University Press, 1993.

JOURNAL ARTICLES

Adashi, Eli Y., H. Jack Geiger, and Michael D. Fine. "Health Care Reform and Primary Care— The Growing Importance of the Community Health Center." *The New England Journal of Medicine*, April 28, 2010.

Beito, David. "Black Fraternal Hospitals of the Mississippi Delta." *The Journal of Southern History* (February 1999): 109–140.

Bethell, Thomas N. "Sumter County Blues: The Ordeal of the Federation of Southern Cooperatives," a report for the National Committee in Support of Community Based Organizations (Washington, D.C., 1982).

Brown, Roy E. "Delivery of Pediatric Health Services in a Rural Health Center." *Pediatrics* 44: 3 (September, 1969): 333–337.

Brown, Thomas and Elizabeth Fee. "Sidney Kark and John Cassel: Social Medicine Pioneers and South African Emigrés." *American Journal of Public Health* 92:11 (November 2002): 1744–1745.

Carter, Luther. "Rural Health: OEO Launches Bold Mississippi Project." *Science* 156 (June 16, 1967): 1466–1468.

Dorsey, L.C. "Harder Times than These." *Southern Exposure* (1982): 28–31.

Geiger, H. J. "A Health Center for Social Change: People and Poverty in Rural Mississippi," Supplementary Text published by *Network for Continuing Medical Education*. New York, June 1971, p. 24.

Geiger, H. Jack. "Community Control—or Community Conflict?" *Bulletin of the National Tuberculosis and Respiratory Disease Association* (November 1969): 4–10.

Geiger, H. Jack. "Community-Oriented Primary Care: The Legacy of Sidney Kark." *American Journal of Public Health*, 83:7 (July 1993): 946–947.

Geiger, H. Jack. "Community-Oriented Primary Care: A Path to Community Development." *American Journal of Public Health* 92: 11 (November 2002): 1713–1716.

Geiger, H. Jack. "The First Community Health Centers: A Model of Enduring Value." *Journal of Ambulatory Care Management* 28: 4 (October–December 2005): 313–320.

Hatch, John W. "Discussion of Group Practice in Comprehensive Healthcare Centers." *Bulletin of the New York Academy of Medicine*. Second series, 44: 11 (November 1968): 1375–1377.

Hansen, Christian. "The Pediatrician and Family Planning in a Very Poor Community: An Appraisal of Experiences in the Tufts Delta Health Ctr., Bolivar County, Mississippi." *Clinical Pediatrics* (June 1972): 319–323.

Huttie, Joseph J. Jr. "New Federalism and the Death of a Dream in Mound Bayou, Mississippi." *New South* 28:4 (Fall 1973): 20–29.

"In Remembrance: Sister Mary Stella Simpson, ACNM's Fifth President." *Journal of Midwifery & Women's Health* (2004): 469.

James, Andrew. "Tufts–Delta Administers Environmental Treatment." *The Journal of Environmental Health* 31: 5 (March–April, 1969): 437–446.

Kelly, Cynthia. "Health Care in the Mississippi Delta." *American Journal of Nursing* 69: 4 (April 1969): 758–763.

Morgan, Bruce. "Up from Mississippi," *Tufts Medicine* 62: 2 (Spring 2003): 16–25.

"Moral Consciousness and Commitment in Mound Bayou." *Meharry Medical College Quarterly Digest* (January 1970): 11–15.

Robinson, Pearl B. "The Community Part in Health Center Program," presented at the 97th Annual Meeting of the American Public Health Association and Meeting of Related Organizations, Nov. 10–14, 1969, Philadelphia, Penn. Excerpted in "Voices from the Past," *American Journal of Public Health* (September 11, 2014): e3.

Walker, Matthew. "The Affiliation of Taborian Hospital with Meharry Medical College and Development of the OEO Planning Grant," *Meharry Medical College Quarterly Digest* 4 (April 1966): 3.

NEWSPAPERS AND NEWSMAGAZINES

"28-Year Partnership for Health in Mississippi," *Ebony* (April 1970): 48, 50, 52.

Bims, Hamilton. "The Neighborhood Center: Newest Public Health Remedy." *Ebony* (Nov. 1970): 124–132.

Black, Herbert. "Destitute Southern Hospital Saved." *The Boston Globe,* May 28, 1974.

Cardon, Justin. "L. C. Dorsey." *Jackson Free Press,* August 26, 2013.

Carter, Hodding. "He's Doing Something About the Race Problem." *Saturday Evening Post* (February 23, 1946): 31.

Cefalu, Laura. "Tufts Center, Mound Bayou hospital clash." *Delta Democrat-Times,* October 19, 1970.

"Center Built Despite Obstacles." Jackson *Clarion-Ledger,* n.d., 2000.

Coates, Ta-Nehisi. "The Case for Reparations." *The Atlantic* (June 2014): 54–71.

Cobb, Carl. "Mississippi Medicine" series. *The Boston Globe,* July 16–20, 1967.

"Delta Health Center Takes Medics to Cotton Turn Rows," Jackson *Clarion-Ledger,* Nov. 14, 1971.

"From Plantation to Law School: She Thinks This Trip is Necessary," *The New York Times,* Feb. 14, 1973.

Hall, Richard. "A Stir of Hope in Mound Bayou." *LIFE* (March 28, 1969): 67–79.

Knox, Richard. "Hope Comes to Mound Bayou." *The Boston Globe,* April 26, 1970.

Lyons, Richard. "Grip of Poverty Chokes Mississippi Children." *Memphis Commercial Appeal,* April 1, 1968.

McGill, Ralph. "Health in Action Areas." *The Daily Reporter* (Dover, Ohio), April 26, 1967, p. 4.

Hansen, Suzy. "What Can Mississippi Learn from Iran?" *The New York Times,* July 27, 2012.

Haskell, David. "Pilot Program: Comprehensive Medical Health Program Proven." *The Daily Herald* (Provo, Utah), April 18, 1968, p. 19.

Letter from "Sad Nurse" to Mr. A. B. Albritton. *Memphis Commercial Appeal,* July 31, 1972.

"Letters to the Editor." *LIFE,* April 18, 1969, p. 22B.

Maxwell, Neil. "The Ailing Poor." *The Wall Street Journal,* January 14, 1969.

McDaniel, C. G. "Community Health Centers More Than Clinics for the Poor." *Arizona Republic,* Sept. 5, 1971.

"Medical Association Head Opposed to Federal Health Unit." *Sunday Republican* (Waterbury, Conn.), Nov. 26, 1965.

"Medicine: Mound Bayou's Crisis," *TIME,* Nov. 25, 1974.

"Medicine: Treating the Poor." *TIME,* Nov. 29, 1968.

Mills, Kay. "Dr. Delta." *Mother Jones,* Jan/Feb 1993.

"Mississippians Protest OEO Plans for Bolivar County Health Center." *Memphis Commercial-Appeal,* February 4, 1966.

"Msgr. John Romaniello." *The New York Times,* October 25, 1985.

"Mound Bayou Hospitals: Veto halts merger." *Delta Democrat-Times* (Greenville, Miss.), June 18, 1972.

The Mound Bayou [Mississippi] *Voice.*

"New Hospital is First Tangible By-Product of Tufts Project." *The Boston Globe,* July 18, 1967.

"OEO Grant set for Mound Bayou." *Delta Democrat-Times* (Greenville, Miss.), July 5, 1970.

UPI, "Comprehensive Health Care for the Needy." *The Bridgeport (Conn.) Post,* April 14, 1968, p.12.

Rose, Bill. "Court Eyes Delta Food." *Delta-Democrat Times* (Greenville, Miss.), March 31, 1971, p. 1.

Rose, Bill. "Many Ways Tried to Salvage DFP." *Delta-Democrat Times* (Greenville, Miss.), March 31, 1971, p. 16.

"Rosedale to get $148,000." *Delta Democrat-Times* (Greenville, Miss.), May 28, 1972.

Reed, Roy. "Equal Service Edict Irks Town." *The New York Times*, March 2, 1971.

Reed, Roy. "Political Dispute Perils Funds for Mississippi Health Facility." *The New York Times*, July 17, 1972.

"Sit and Die for Lack of $3." *Boston Globe*, July 17, 1967.

Taylor, Owen. "Duncan Invisible Boycott." *Delta Democrat-Times* (Greenville, Miss.), September 5, 1971.

Taylor, Owen. "Mississippi, Meet the Noodle." *Delta Democrat-Times* (Greenville, Miss.), Nov. 11, 1971.

"To Rural Negroes, Health Care is Hope." *The New York Times,* August 28, 1970.

Tong, Hiram. "The Pioneers of Mound Bayou." *The Century Magazine* (1908): 390–400.

"Tufts Plan: Negroes' Only Ray of Hope." *Boston Globe*, July 16, 1967.

The Taborian Star (Cary, Mississippi), March 1942.

"Waller OK's Health Grant; Calls Bayou Project 'Fiasco'." *Memphis Commercial Appeal*, July 8, 1972.

"We Need More Doctors," *Jet* (Feb. 15, 1973): 30–31.

"Where Everything's Fine." *St. Louis Post-Dispatch*, March 30, 1968.

THESES AND DISSERTATIONS

Sobelson, Morissa G. "Participation, Power, and Place: Roots of the Community Health Center Movement." Honors thesis, Tufts University, 2009.

Howard, S. J., and Paul Francis. "Report of a Work Project in the Environmental Services Division of Tufts-Delta Health Center, Mound Bayou, Mississippi." M.S. Thesis in Environmental Health Engineering, Tufts University, May 1971.

WEBSITES

Edelman, Marian Wright. "Still Hungry in America." *The Huffington Post*, Feb. 2, 2102. http://www.huffingtonpost.com/marian-wright-edelman/hunger-in-america_b_1269450.html#es_share_ended.

Geiger, H. Jack. "Voting is Good for Your Health!" Guest blog, Campaign for America's Health Centers, March 12, 2102 http://blog.saveourchcs.org/2012/03/29/voting-is-good-for-your-health

Health Resources & Services Administration Fact Sheet. http://bphc.hrsa.gov/about/health-centerfactsheet.pdf

Mississippi Primary Health Care Association. "Community Health Centers Directory of Services, 2011." www.mphca.com/313047+MPHCA-Directory+of+Services+2011.pdf.

National Association of Community Health Centers. "United States Health Center Fact Sheet." https://www.nachc.com/client/documents/America's_CHCs1014.pdf.

Rutherford, Karen. "L. C. Dorsey." *The Mississippi Writers Page.* http://www.olemiss.edu/mwp/dir/dorsey_lc/.

Thomas-Tisdale, Alice. "Legacy of L. C. Dorsey is Unparalleled in the War on Poverty in Mississippi." *Jackson Advocate* (http://www.jacksonadvocateonline.com/?p=10548.

U.S. National Library of Medicine. "Community Health: A Model for the World," in *Against the Odds: Making a Difference in Global Health*. http://apps.nlm.nih.gov/againsttheodds/ exhibit/community_health/model_world.cfm.

Varney, Sarah. "How Obamacare Went South in Mississippi." *Kaiser Health News,* October 29, 2014. http://khn.org/news/how-obamacare-went-south-in-mississippi/.

INDEX